• • •

"IT'S NOT WHAT WE DO ONCE IN A WHILE
THAT SHAPES OUR LIVES, BUT WHAT WE
DO CONSISTENTLY."

• • •

TONY ROBBINS

CONTENT

• • •

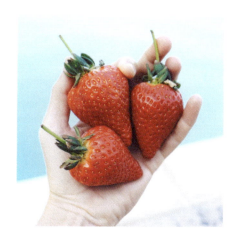
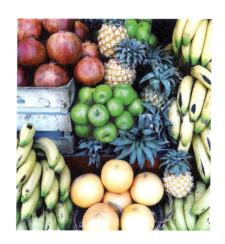

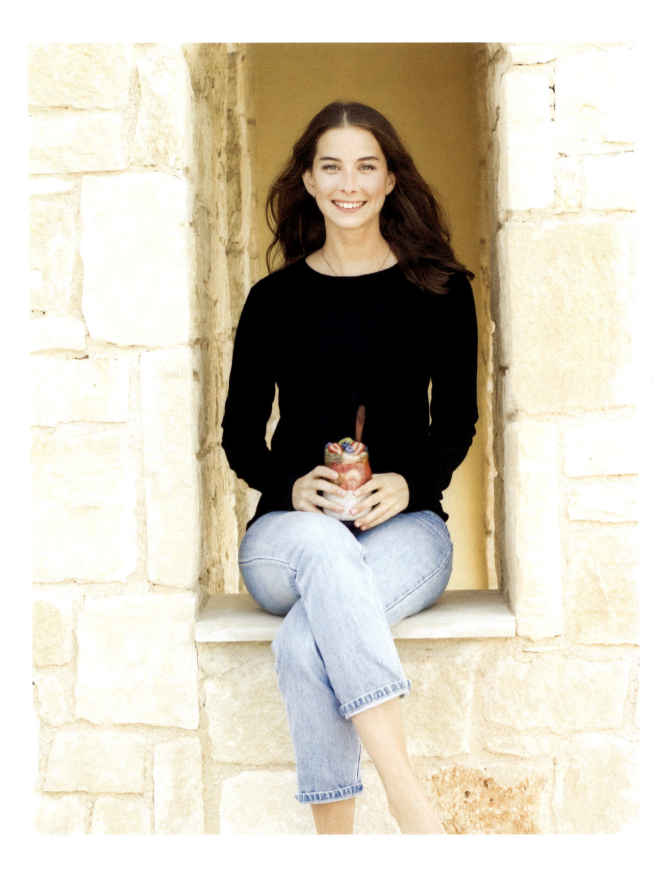

SOMETHING SWEET

• • •

Cakes, ice cream, cookies, puddings, candy, oh my! Sweet desserts are a temptation that can be hard to resist, even for the most health-conscious among us. How many times did we start a new 'diet' accompanied with terrible guilt feelings about treating ourselves, as we'd fear this might undo all of the hard work (yes, we have all been there)? Many 'diets' out there promote some sort of calorie restriction, including the reduction of fruits and carbohydrates, leaving you bouncing back and forth with on/off dieting. Treating yourself is important - we all enjoy eating our favorite sweet treat. It not only satisfies our natural sweet tooth but also relieves our bodies and minds from intense cravings.

After 10 years of struggling with unsuccessful diets, self-love, binging, and health-issues I have finally found something to ground me and enable a positive relationship between food and my body, leaving me with the desire to become the best and healthiest version of myself. Instead of promoting short-term weight loss, I am promoting a long-term lifestyle that will enable you to reach your optimum health and body weight. We all wish to live a healthy and well balanced life. In

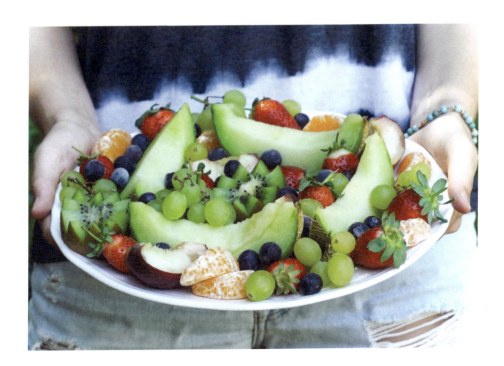

contrast to numerous 'quick fixes', I am a big proponent of a sustainable wholefoods plant-based approach, including the occasional treat. Most desserts, however, are loaded with dairy, eggs, fats and sugars. Even many vegan options out there are full of added refined sugars, processed ingredients and oils.

Combining the desire for sweets with a balaced healthy lifestyle, this book is all about enjoying 'clean' wholesome treats without feeling bad about it - in other words, healthy and tasty food that let's your body thrive! That's why it was important that all the sweets included would be plant-based, refined sugar-free, oil-free, partly gluten-free and be made with natural ingredients only that are 100% nutritious. Don't judge a book by its cover - these desserts will leave you wanting seconds!

A healthy lifestyle can not only help you get in shape, but also make you you feel better and lead a happier life. Although it sounds fairly simple, the path there can be very challenging. No matter if you are just starting out or have been doing it for years, don't be too hard on yourself and don't let others discourage you! You have the power to make the conscious decision of caring for your body every single day. I hope this book will inspire and motivate you on your journey to health and happiness. Because, ultimately, that's what it's all about.

• • •

Kirsten
♡

PLANT-BASED

Plant foods are the healthiest food on this planet. They are not only a great source of energy but also have the power to heal our bodies and reverse/prevent diseases. They are packed with fiber, vitamins, minerals and healthy fats, which our bodies need to thrive. A diet consisiting of vegetables, fruits, legumes and nuts & seeds is not only extremely nutritious but also really satisfying to our bodies.

NO REFINED SUGAR

Refined and processed sugars, such as table sugar, high fructose corn syrup and agave syrup, are considered 'empty calories', which have been stripped of almost all fiber, vitamins and minerals. These empty carbs digest much quicker than whole foods and have a high glycemic index, which leads to rapid spikes in blood sugar and insulin levels. Many studies link the consumption of refined sugars with a drastically increased risk of diseases (obesity, heart disease, etc.) and inflammation, suggesting that refined sugars are toxic for our bodies. There are, however, alternative sweeteners, which are much healthier. Using natural sweeteners, such as whole fruits, molasses, date & maple syrup, not only satisfies our sweet tooth but also provides an unrefined and nutritionally beneficial alternative.

OIL-FREE

Oil is the most calorie dense food. With 120 calories per tablespoon, it is twice as calorie rich as refined sugar. Despite common belief, vegetable oils are not a health or weight-loss food. Although olive and coconut oil are often labelled as 'good fats', this description is only true compared to animal fats. Similar to refined sugar, oils have almost completely been stripped of fiber, vitamins and minerals. Hence, oils are not only highly processed but also offer very few nutritional benefits for our bodies.

Coconut oil, in particular, consist of 90% saturated fat and has shown to worsen bad cholesterol levels. While I do consume oils from time to time, I try not to introduce them as a regular part of my diet. Not to worry though, cooking and baking without oils is fairly easy once you know how. In baking, oil can usually be replaced with mashed bananas, apple sauce or nut milks that are higher in good fat. In cooking, simply use non-sticking pans and a dash of vegetable broth to sauté onions and garlic. These simple tips really helped me to significantly reduce the amount of extra calories and unhealthy saturated fats in my diet.

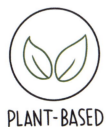

PLANT-BASED

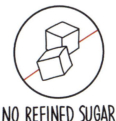

NO REFINED SUGAR

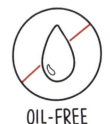

OIL-FREE

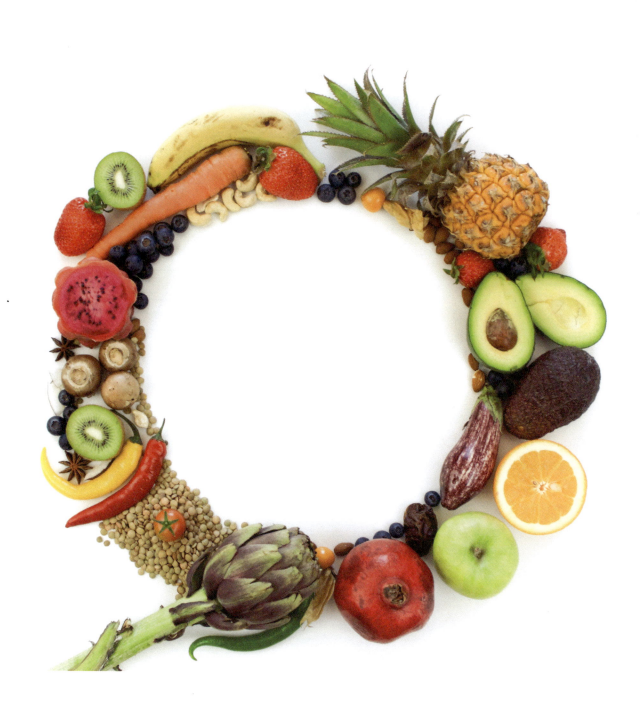

MEASUREMENTS

All recipes in this book use the standard American cup system (240ml) of measuring ingredients by volume. Measuring cups are widely available and very easy to use. In case you do not have access to measuring cups, or simply prefer the metric or imperial system, I have included a conversion chart below.

US cups	Metric	Imperial
1 Tbsp	15ml	1/2fl oz
1/8 cup	30ml	1fl oz
1/4 cup	60ml	2fl oz
1/3 cup	75ml	2-1/2fl oz
1/2 cup	120ml	4fl oz
3/4 cup	180ml	6fl oz
1 cup	240ml	8fl oz

EQUIPMENT

Aside from standard sized staple baking tins and utensils, the only thing I swear by in the kitchen is a good quality high-speed blender (I use the Optimum 9200A). It will allow you to make super creamy, smooth frostings, cake crusts and cookies in no time! Any extra equipment for specific desserts (e.g. ice cream molds) can be found on my website www.thetastyk.com/equipment.

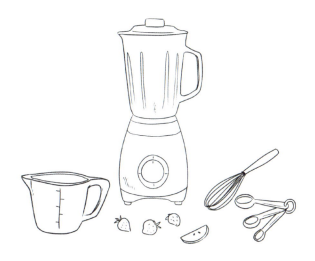

INGREDIENTS

• • •

This book is all about simplifying healthy plant-based cooking. That is why the focus is on using natural ingredients that are commonly available in grocery and health food stores around the world. The majority of the ingredients and methods should be familiar to you, but if you are new to the plant-based kitchen, there may be a few ingredients you haven't heard of before.

MEDJOOL DATES

Medjool dates are a specific type of the date fruit, originating from North Africa and the Middle East. They are prized for their large size, sweet caramel-like taste and juicy flesh. You can find them in most health food stores or buy them in bulk online.

GROUND VANILLA BEANS

Vanilla beans ground to a fine powder are very exquisite and flavorful as they are not diluted by alcohol. Hence, you won't lose any flavor when cooking or baking with ground vanilla beans.

CACAO VS. COCOA POWDER

Numerous studies have shown the nutritional benefits of consuming cacao/cocoa. It is loaded with antioxidants, vitamins and can lower your blood pressure, insulin resistance and risk of stroke. There are two different powders commonly available. Cacao powder is made by cold-pressing unroasted cocoa beans, which keeps the living enyzmes and removes the fat. Cocoa powder is raw cacao that has been roast-

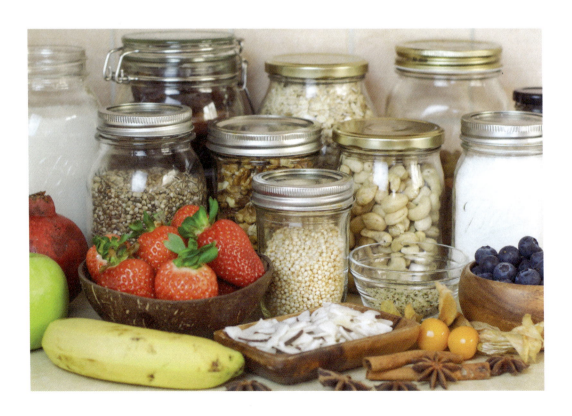

ed at high temperatures, which reduces the enzyme content and overall nutritional value. While raw cacao powder is nutritionally more beneficial and less processed, it is also much more expensive. Whichever variety you end up using, make sure that it is plain without added sugars, milk fats or oil. In many countries the cocoa powder you can buy in supermarkets has these added components to overcome the acidic nature and bitter taste.

Both cacao and cocoa are highly nutritious and will surely satisfy your chocolate cravings.

FLAX EGGS

Flax eggs serve as an egg replacement in baking. 1 flax egg consists of 1 Tbsp ground flaxseeds (flaxmeal) and 2-3 Tbsp water. Simply combine both ingredients in a small bowl and let them soak for 5-10 minutes. The flaxseeds will absorb the water and form a sticky egg-like substance.

DARK VEGAN CHOCOLATE

Contrary to popular belief, not all dark chocolate is vegan. Some dark chocolates include whey or non-fat milk powder so make sure to always check the label. Usually, the higher the cocoa percentage the healthier and the more chances it will be vegan (75-90%).

SOAKED CASHEWS

Soaking cashews or nuts in general helps break down the enzyme inhibitors. This will ease digestion and enhance nutrient absorbtion. Simply place the nuts in a bowl, cover them com-pletely with filtered water and let them soak overnight (7-24 hours). Drain and rinse them properly before using in your favorite recipes.

COCONUT CREAM

Coconut cream is very similar to coconut milk. However, it is different in consistency and contains less water. The cream is made from 4 parts coconut meat and 1 part water (in comparison to 1:1), which yields a rich and creamy paste-like result. Hence, coconut cream is higher in fat and calories. When buying canned coconut cream/milk, the inside is usually liquid. If you place the can in the fridge overnight, the creamy part will separate from the liquid and form a thick paste on the top of the can, which can be used in baking or cooking. The brand is important. Some milks just don't separate no matter how long they are stored in the fridge, so you'll have to try out a couple of different brands to see which ones work.

NATURAL PEANUT BUTTER

Natural peanut butter usually consists of only one or two ingredients (roasted peanuts and a bit of sea salt). With any store-bought nut butters you want to make sure to purchase the ones with the least amount of ingredients. There is no need for added oils (especially palm oil), refined sugars or any ingredients you cannot pronounce. If you don't want to rely on store-bought versions and have a high quality blender, you'll find it fairly easy to make your own at home.

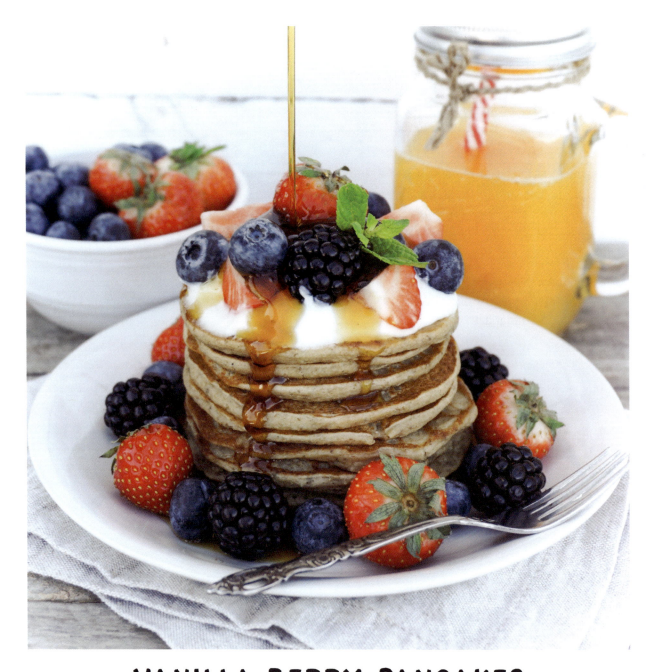

» VANILLA BERRY PANCAKES «

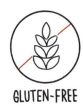

GLUTEN-FREE

serves 2

PANCAKES

1 cup oat flour

1 ripe banana

1 cup almond milk

1 Tbsp chia seeds

1 tsp vanilla extract

1 tsp baking powder

TOPPINGS

Coconut yogurt

Maple syrup

Fresh berries (strawberries, blueberries, blackberries)

Regular pancakes made with white flour, milk, eggs and white sugar can be very heavy and fattening, since they are loaded with empty carbs. These pancakes, in contrast, are naturally sweetened, gluten-free (optional), whole grain, egg-free, and most importantly satisfying. They are incredibly tasty and will have you hooked at first bite!

1. Place the ripe banana in a medium sized bowl and mash it with a fork.

2. Add the remaining ingredients to the bowl and combine.

3. Heat up a non-sticking pan and pour in the batter, forming small pancakes. Once you see bubbles forming flip them over.

4. Top with coconut yogurt, berries and maple syrup and enjoy!

> **TiP HOW TO MAKE OAT FLOUR**
> Simply place the rolled oats into your blender and pulse a few times. If you want to save time you can also just place all ingredients in your blender and voilà! Keep in mind that the batter will thicken as it sits. Add more liquid if needed.

13

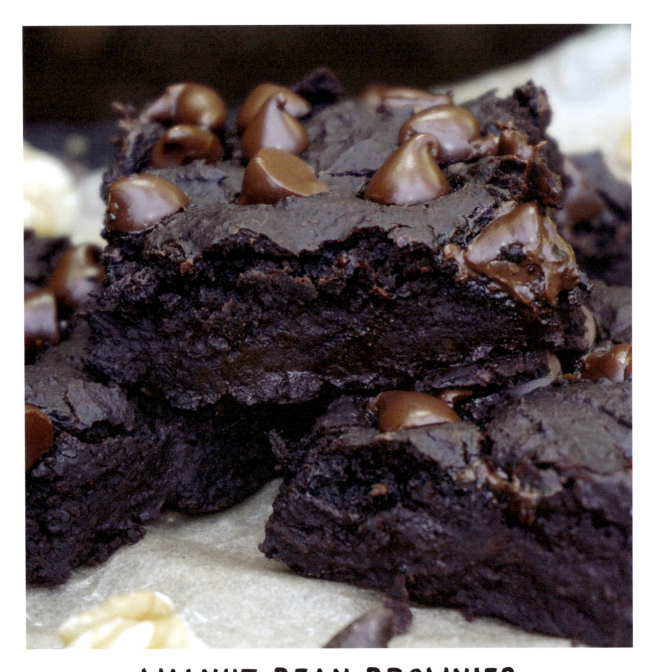

» WALNUT BEAN BROWNIES «

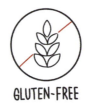

GLUTEN-FREE

◇◇◇◇◇◇◇◇◇◇◇◇◇◇◇◇◇◇◇◇◇◇◇◇◇◇◇

BROWNIES

1 can kidney or black beans
(14oz can)

1/2 cup cacao powder

1 cup Medjool dates, pitted

2 'flax eggs' (combine 2 Tbsp
ground flax seeds + 6 Tbsp
water)

1/3 cup walnuts

1/4 cup almond milk

1 tsp vanilla extract

1 tsp baking powder

3-4 Tbsp dark vegan chocolate
chips (optional)

These walnut bean brownies are a true winner. They are not only extremely delicious but also refined sugar-free, oil-free and gluten-free. The beans not only replace the flour from conventional brownies, but, at the same time, jam-pack this treat with protein and vitamins!

◇◇◇◇◇◇◇◇◇◇◇◇◇◇◇◇◇◇◇◇◇◇◇◇◇◇◇◇◇◇◇◇◇◇◇◇◇◇◇

1. Preheat the oven to 175°C/350°F. Prepare the flax eggs and drain and rinse the kidney beans.

2. Place the beans and the rest of the ingredients (except for the chocolate chips) in a high-speed blender and mix until combined.

3. Line a brownie tin (8"x8") with parchment paper and pour in the dough mixture. Spread the dough evenly and place the chocolate chips on top.

4. Bake for about 30 minutes at 175°C/350°F and let cool down before cutting into squares.

NOTE

For this recipe I used a 8" x 8" (20cm x 20cm) square cake tin.

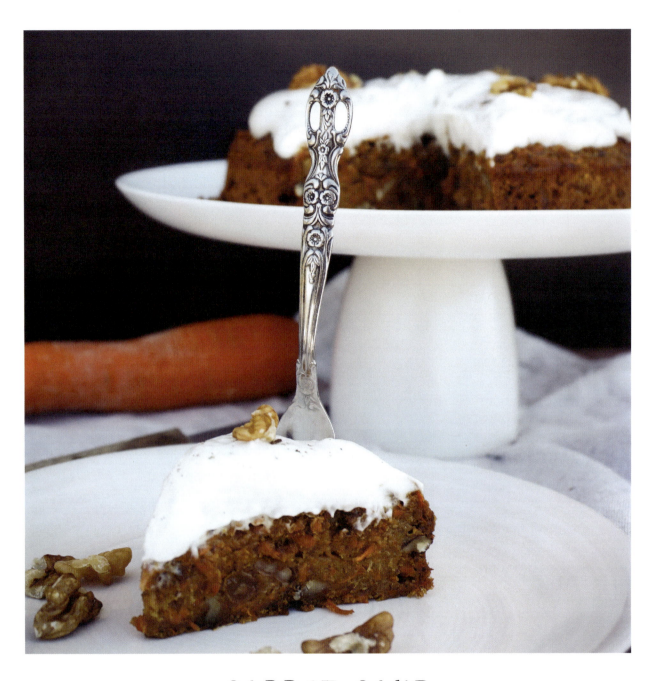

» CARROT CAKE «

WITH COCONUT WHIPPED CREAM

CAKE

3 cups carrots, grated

1 1/2 cups spelt flour

1/2 cup walnuts, chopped

1 1/2 cups almond milk

2 Tbsp ground flax seeds

1 Tbsp vanilla extract

1 tsp baking powder

1/2 cup Medjool dates, pitted and chopped

1 tsp cinnamon, ginger and 1/2 tsp nutmeg

1/3 cup raisins (optional)

WHIPPED CREAM

1 can (15oz) full fat coconut cream (the solid part)

1 Tbsp maple syrup

1/2 tsp vanilla extract

Carrot cake is everybody's favorite, am I right? That's why it can't be missing in this dessert collection! This version is not only plant-based, but also super flavorful, incredibly delicious and guilt-free! Top the cake with delicious coconut whipped cream and enjoy!

1. Grate the carrots, place them in a big bowl and preheat the oven to 175°C/350°F.

2. Add the flour, spices, baking powder, flax seeds and walnuts to the bowl and mix together

3. Add the remaining ingredients and combine with a spatula until your dough is thoroughly mixed.

4. Place the dough into a cake tin (8"/20cm) and place the tin in the oven for 60 minutes or until a toothpick comes out clean.

5. In the meantime, make the coconut whipped cream by placing all ingredients into a bowl and whisking them up with a hand mixer. Place in the fridge until the cake is ready and cooled.

> **TiP   HOW TO MAKE COCO WHIPPED CREAM**
>
> Place a can of full fat coconut cream in the fridge overnight. Due to the high fat percentage, the cream will form up on the top of the can, ready to use for delicious whipped cream!

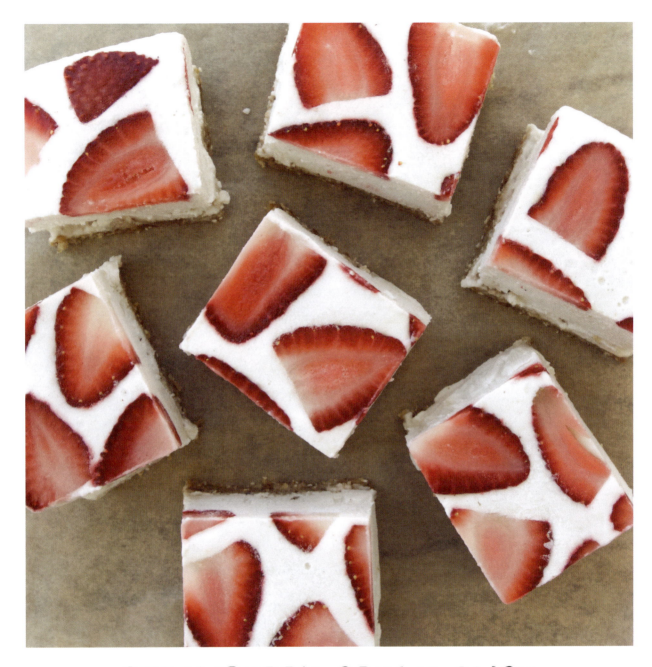

» STRAWBERRY CREAM SLICE «

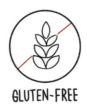

GLUTEN-FREE

CRUST

1 cup rolled oats

1/2 cup walnuts

8 Medjool dates, pitted

Dash of water (optional)

FILLING

1 1/2 cups raw cashews (soaked for min. 6 hours)

1 can (15oz) full fat coconut cream

1/3 cup maple syrup

1 tsp vanilla bean powder

TOPPING

Strawberries, sliced

This delicious strawberry cream slice is not only very eye pleasing but also tastes divine! With 8 ingredients only it is super simple to make and for sure a crowd please. No complicated ingredients, no time wasted in the kitchen! The perfect cool treat to enjoy during summer or just anytime!

1. Place all the crust ingredients into a high-speed blender or food processor and blend until you have a sticky dough.

2. Line a square cake tin with parchment paper and press down the dough evenly. Place in the freezer.

3. In the meantime, make the filling. Simply place all ingredients into a high-speed blender and mix until smooth.

4. Pour the filling over the crust layer and spread evenly. Place the sliced strawberries inside and on top of the filling and place back into the freezer for 5-6 hours (or until firm).

5. Let the cake defrost at room temperature before cutting and serving.

NOTE

For this recipe I used a 8″ x 8″ (20cm x 20cm) square cake tin.

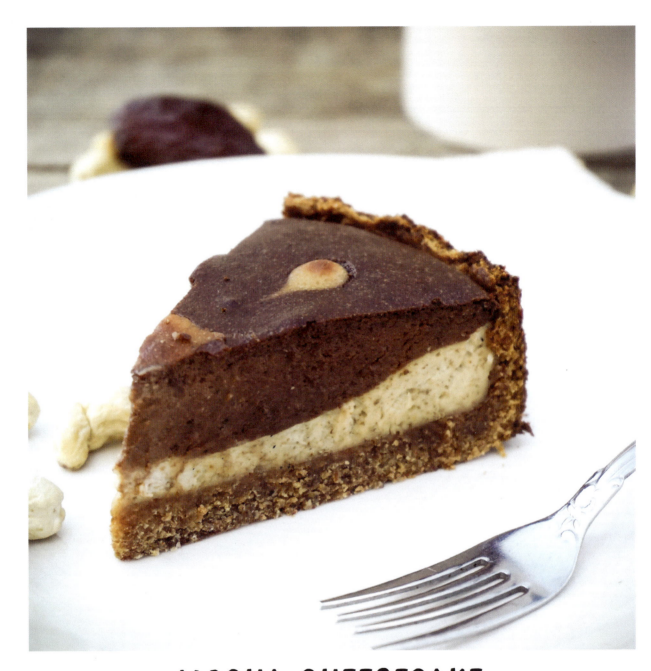

» MOCHA CHEESECAKE «

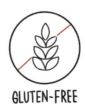

GLUTEN-FREE

serves 10-12

CRUST

1 cup oat flour

1/4 cup walnuts

2 Tbsp instant mocha coffee

1 cup Medjool dates, pitted

1 tsp vanilla extract

A pinch of Himalayan salt

FILLING

1 cup raw cashews (soaked for
min. 6 hours)

300gr soy/ coconut yoghurt

1/3 cup maple syrup

1.5 Tbsp chia seeds

1 tsp vanilla extract
• • • • •
1 Tbsp cacao powder

1/8 cup instant mocha coffee

2 Tbsp maple syrup

Baked cheesecake is a classic! This mocha-vanilla layered version is a must-try for all the coffee & cheesecake lovers out there. It's not only super creamy and delicious, but also really healthy!

1. Preheat the oven to 175°C/350°F.

2. Place the crust ingredients into a high-speed blender/ food processor and blend until you get a crumbly dough.

3. Grease a cake tin and evenly press down the dough into the bottom and sides.

4. Place the first 5 filling ingredients in a high-speed blender and blend them up until smooth.

5. Pour half of the filling into the cake tin.

6. Add cacao powder, instant coffee and 2 Tbsp of maple syrup to the remaining part and blend them up.

7. Carefully pour the mocha filling on top of the other and place in the oven for 40-45 minutes (if you want, use a toothpick to create pretty swirls).

NOTE

For this recipe I used a 8″ (20cm) round cake tin.

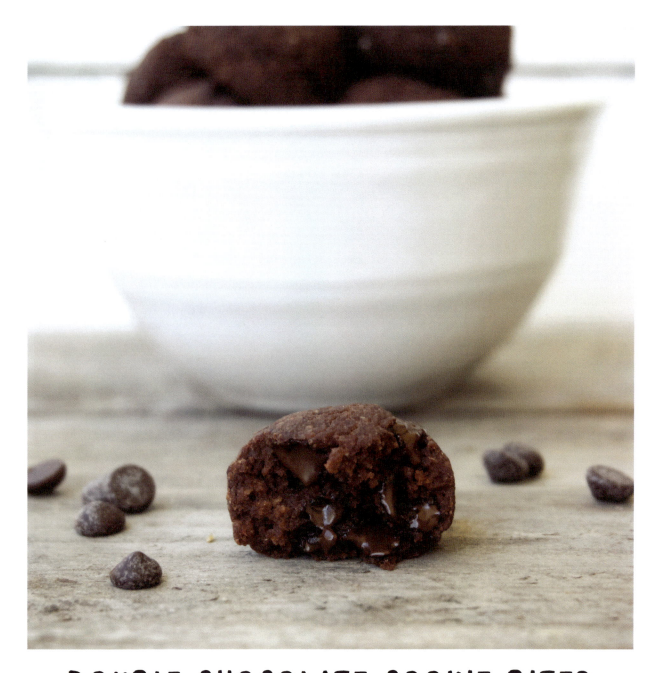

» DOUBLE CHOCOLATE COOKIE BITES «

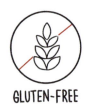

GLUTEN-FREE

serves 20

◇◇◇◇◇◇◇◇◇◇◇◇◇◇◇◇◇◇◇◇◇◇◇◇◇◇◇◇◇

1 can kidney beans (15oz),
drained and rinsed

1/2 cup oat flour

1/3 cup natural almond butter,
melted

1/8 cup almond milk

1/4 cup date syrup

1/3 cup cacao powder

1 tsp baking powder

• • • • •

1/3 cup dark vegan chocolate
chips

As part of my healthy cookie bites series these delicious double chocolate cookies will leave you wanting more! Jam-packed with protein, these little bundles of joy have a soft core with melted chocolate and are slightly crunchy on the outside. They are not only the perfect healthy go-to snack but also kid-friendly!

◇◇◇

1. Preheat the oven to 175°C/350°F and line a baking tray with parchment paper.

2. Place the first 7 ingredients in your high-speed blender/ food processor and use the blender stick to mash them down until you have a more or less smooth batter.

3. Place the batter in a bowl, add in the chocolate chips and combine with a spatula.

4. Use your hands to form small bite-sized balls and place on the baking tray.

5. Place the tray in the oven and bake for 10-15 minutes.

> **TiP HEALTH BENEFITS OF KIDNEY BEANS**
>
> Kidney beans, like other legumes, are extremely high in protein and fiber, and also contain numerous vitamins and minerals. They are particularly high in molybdenum, iron and folate.

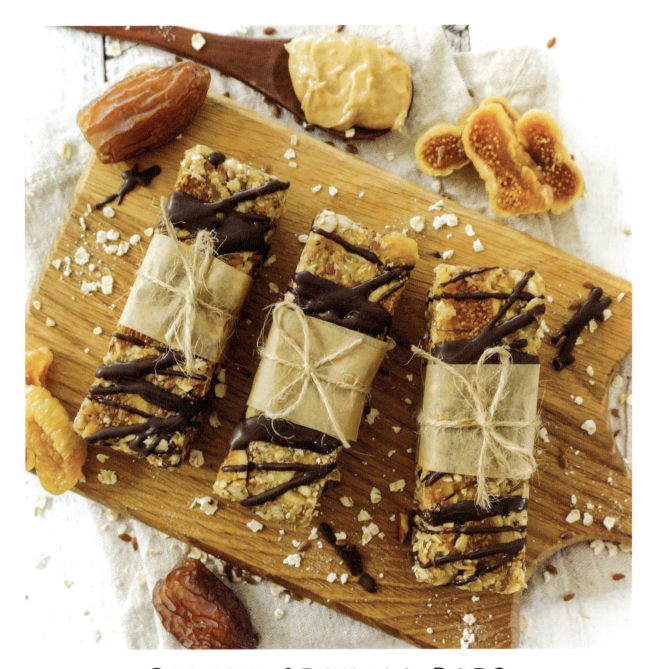

» PEANUT GRANOLA BARS «

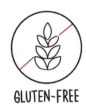

GLUTEN-FREE

serves 8

◇◇

INGREDIENTS

10 Medjool dates, pitted

2 cups rolled oats

1/2 cup dried figs, sliced

2 Tbsp chia seeds

3 Tbsp flax seeds

3 Tbsp desiccated coconut

2 Tbsp almonds, chopped

1 tsp ground vanilla bean

1 Tbsp natural peanut butter

3 Tbsp sunflower seeds

1/2 cup water (more if needed)

TOPPINGS

1/4 cup melted dark vegan chocolate

Granola bars are an amazing snack! They're just perfect to bring to any occasion, may it be the office, hikes, or before workouts. Unfortunately, most store-bought granola bars are loaded with added sugars. These super easy peanut granola bars, in contrast, are healthy, full of wholesome ingredients and naturally sweetened with dates.

◇◇

1. Place the dates into a high-speed blender or food processor. Add a dash of water and blend until you have a smooth date paste.

2. Add the date paste and all other remaining ingredients to a bowl and knead together with your hands.

3. Once combined, press the mixture into a square baking tin (lined with parchment paper) and place into the freezer for 30 minutes.

4. Once firm, drizzle melted dark vegan chocolate on top and let dry. Cut into bars and store in the fridge/freezer.

NOTE

For this recipe I used a regular bread loaf baking tin. Any similar rectangular tin would work.

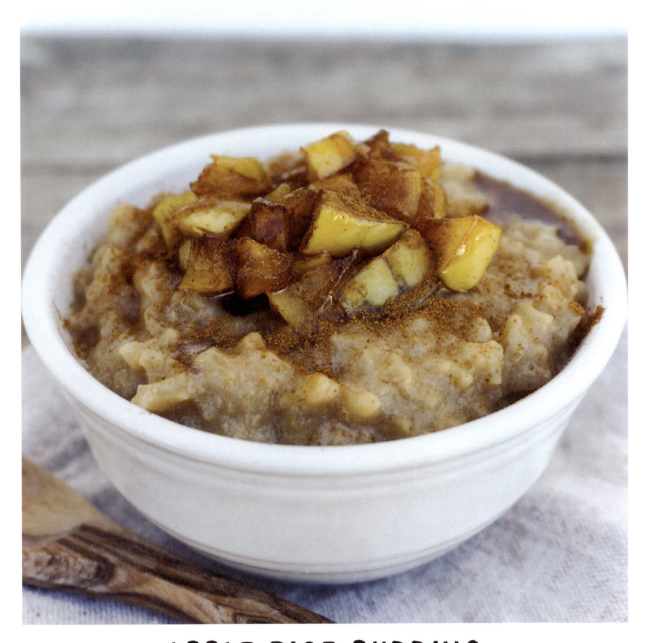

» APPLE RICE PUDDING «

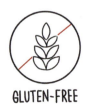

GLUTEN-FREE

serves 2

INGREDIENTS

2 cups almond milk

3/4 cup water

1/3 cup short grain white rice

2 Tbsp maple syrup

1/2 tsp vanilla extract

1 tsp lemon zest

TOPPINGS

1 apple, cut into pieces

1/2 tsp cinnamon

1 Tbsp maple syrup

Rice pudding can be found on dessert menus across many countries. Essentially there are two ways of preparing rice pudding, boiling and baking. Most rice puddings are filled with heavy cream, tons of refined sugar and unnecessary fats. This version, however, is much simpler, lower in fat and sugar, so that you can enjoy every bite without feeling guilty.

1. Combine the rice and water in a large saucepan.
2. Bring to a simmer and then reduce the heat to low. Cover and let simmer until the water has been absorbed.
3. Add the maple syrup, lemon zest, vanilla and almond milk and cook (uncovered) for 30 minutes. Make sure to stir once in a while.
4. Once the milk has been absorbed, remove from the heat and place the rice pudding into small serving bowls.
5. Place the topping ingredients in a small pan and heat up until you have a sticky, cooked apple mixture. Add to the rice pudding and enjoy!

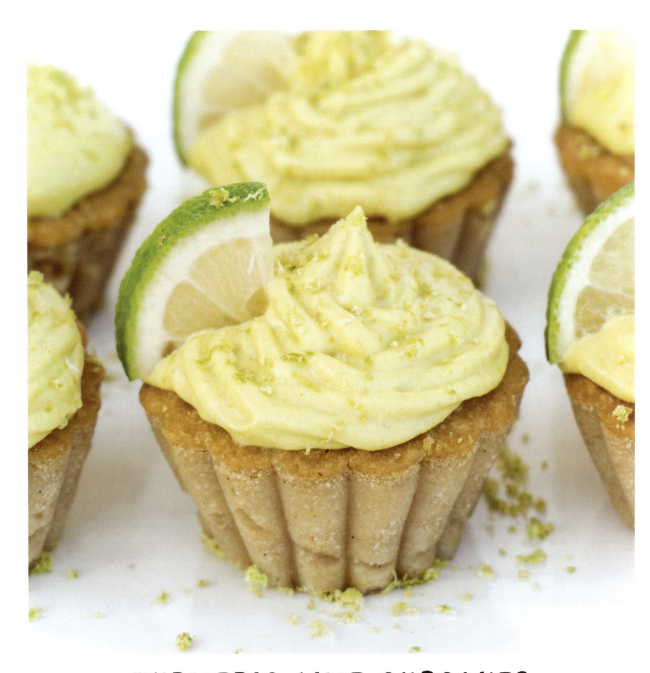

» TURMERIC LIME CUPCAKES «

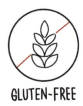

GLUTEN-FREE

serves 6

INGREDIENTS

1 cup rice flour

1/2 cup oat flour

1/2 cup lime juice

1 Tbsp grated lime zest

1 1/3 cup coconut milk

1/4 cup maple syrup

1 tsp vanilla extract

1 tsp baking powder

Pinch of sea salt

FROSTING

1/2 cup cashews, soaked overnight

1/8 cup coconut cream

1/8 cup maple syrup

2 Tbsp lime juice

1 tsp turmeric powder

1/2 tsp vanilla extract

These delicious cupcakes are loaded with fresh citrus flavor, both in the cake and cashew cream frosting! They can be made gluten-free, are incredibly light and super tasty, which makes them the perfect treat for warm summer days!

1. Preheat the oven to 175°C/350°F.
2. Place the dry ingredients into one bowl, whisk together and do the same with the liquid ones. Slowly mix the dry and liquid mixtures together until you have a smooth batter.
3. Pour the batter into cupcake molds and bake in the oven for 25-30 minutes (until toothpick comes out clean).
4. In the meantime, place all frosting ingredients in a high-speed blender and blend until smooth. Store in the fridge. Once the cupcakes are cooled down, use a pipping bag to apply the frosting. Sprinkle lime zest on top and enjoy!

> **TiP** **HEALTH BENEFITS OF TURMERIC**
>
> Turmeric is considered to be 'the queen of spices' with powerful antioxidant and anti-inflammatory properties. Loaded with healthy nutrients like protein, vitamins, calcium and niacin, it is arguably the most powerful herb on the planet at fighting and reversing diseases.

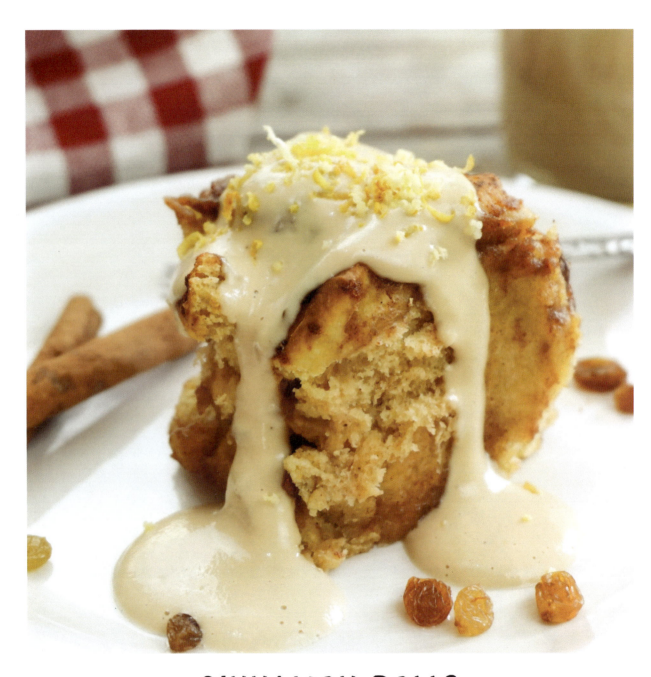

» CINNAMON ROLLS «

WITH LEMON CASHEW CREAM GLAZE

◇◇◇◇◇◇◇◇◇◇◇◇◇◇◇◇◇◇◇◇◇◇◇◇◇◇◇◇◇◇◇

DOUGH

3 cups spelt flour

3/4 cup sweet potato purée

1 cup full fat coconut cream, melted and warmed to the touch

1/4 cup maple syrup

2 tsp instant yeast

Dash of sea salt

FILLING

10 Medjool dates, pitted

1/3 cup rice milk

1 Tbsp ground cinnamon

1/4 cup raisins

GLAZE

1/2 cup cashews, soaked over-night

1/4 cup rice milk

1/8 cup maple syrup

juice of 1/2 a lemon

1. Place a sieve above a bowl and add the flour. Put all the flour through the sieve, add the salt and yeast and combine.

2. In a separate bowl, add the sweet potato purée, maple syrup and warmed coconut cream and combine. Add the liquid to the dry ingredients and combine with a spatula. When it gets too tough, use your hands and knead the dough for 10 minutes (set a timer).

3. Place the dough into a slightly oiled bowl, cover with a kitchen towel and let rest at room temperature for 1-1.5 hours (the dough should have doubled by now).

4. In the meantime, add the dates, cinnamon and milk into a high-speed blender until smooth.

6. Preheat the oven to 175°C/350°F.

7. Once the dough is ready, place it on a floured surface and use a rolling pin to spread the dough evenly into a rectangle. Spread the date filling on top (make sure it's not too thick or it will be difficult to roll) and add some raisins or blueberries. Starting at the longer side of the dough, use your hands to rolls it up (it doesn't matter if it doesn't come out as a perfect roll).

8. Cut the roll into equal pieces and place filling-up into a lined cake tin. Place the tin into the oven and bake for 40-45 minutes (take a toothpick to check if the roll in the middle is baked).

9. In the meantime prepare the glaze by simply blending up all ingredients.

10. Once ready, take out a warm cinnamon roll, top with the glaze, sprinkle some lemon zest on top and enjoy!

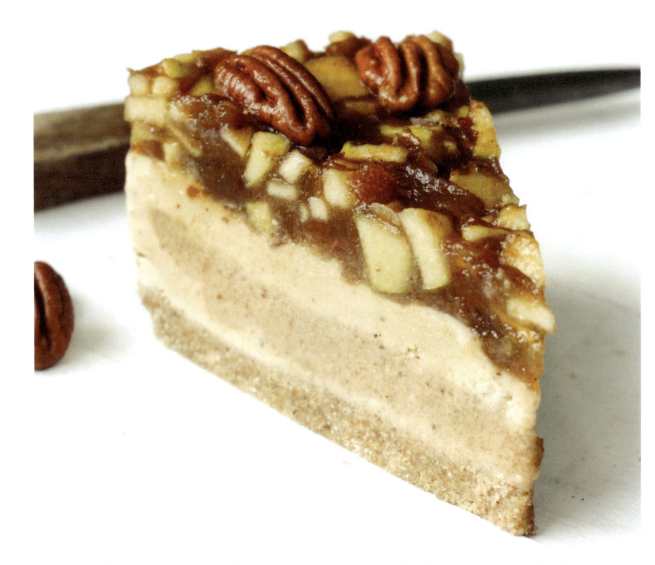

» PECAN APPLE ICE CREAM CAKE «

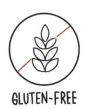

GLUTEN-FREE

CRUST

1/2 cup oat flour

1/2 cup desiccated coconut

1 cup Medjool dates, pitted

1/2 tsp cinnamon

2 Tbsp water

ICE CREAM FILLING

1 cup full-fat coconut cream

1/8 cup maple syrup

1 cup cashews, soaked overnight

1 tsp vanilla extract

CARAMEL LAYER

1 cup Medjool dates, pitted

1/4 cup natural pecans

1/2 cup rice milk

APPLE LAYER

1 cup Medjool dates, pitted

2 apples, diced

1/8 cup water

This decadent pecan apple ice cream cake is the perfect treat to impress family & friends! It's incredibly creamy, flavorful and, best of all, naturally sweetened by nature's sugah! Every bite will melt in your mouth - so yummy!

1. Place all the crust ingredients in a high-speed blender until combined. Press into a cake tin (8" or 20cm) and place in the freezer.

2. Add all ice cream ingredients into the blender and mix for 2-3 minutes. Divide the filling into two equal parts and set aside.

3. Combine all caramel ingredients in the blender and mix until smooth. Pour the first part of the cheesecake filling over the crust and place back into the freezer.

4. After 30 minutes (or until firm), gently spread the caramel layer on top and place it back into the freezer for 10 minutes. Pour the other half on top of the caramel layer and place back into the freezer for 1 hour.

5. Blend up the dates and water until you get a sticky mixture and place it into a bowl. Add the diced apples and whisk it together. Once the cake is firm, gently spread the apple layer on top and place it back into the freezer for 15 minutes. Let defrost at room temperature before eating!

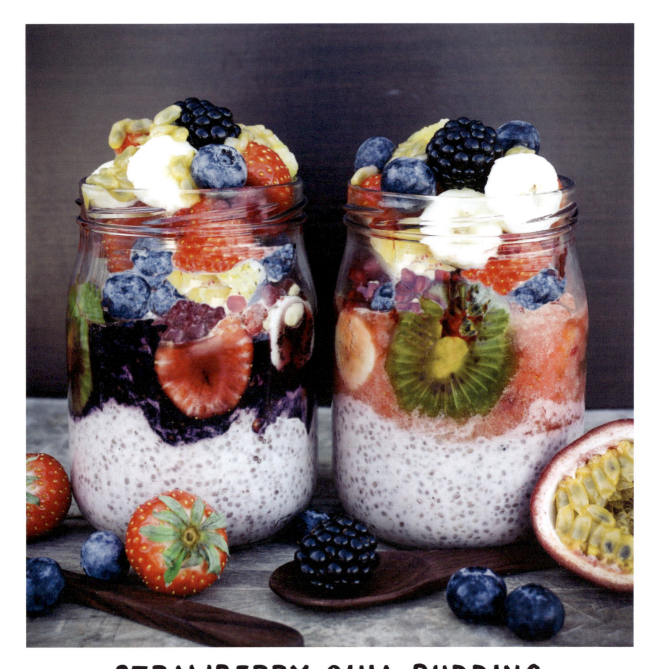

» STRAWBERRY CHIA PUDDING «

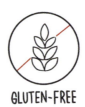

GLUTEN-FREE

serves 2

INGREDIENTS

1/3 cup chia seeds

1 cup coconut milk

1 cup strawberries (fresh or frozen

1/2 tsp vanilla extract

1/8 cup maple syrup

BERRY LAYER

1/2 cup fresh berries (blackberries or strawberries)

1 Tbsp maple syrup

TOPPINGS

Fresh fruit

Chia pudding is an easy and delicious way of taking advantage of the nutritious chia seed. Chia seeds absorb water up to 9 times their weight when soaked, meaning you can use them to make creamy, dreamy pudding!

1. Place all the chia pudding ingredients into a high-speed blender and mix until combined.

2. Divide the pudding into two serving bowls/ glasses and place in the fridge for a minimum of 2 hours (or overnight).

3. For the berry layer, simply add the desired berries with the maple syrup into a blender and mix until smooth.

4. Once the pudding is ready, pour the berry layer on top and decorate with fresh fruit.

TiP HEALTH BENEFITS OF CHIA SEEDS

Chia seeds are a powerhouse of healthy nutrients. They are not only packed with omega-3 fatty acids, but are also high in fiber, protein and antioxidants. Studies suggest that grinding chia seeds helps the body reap greater benefits from the seeds.

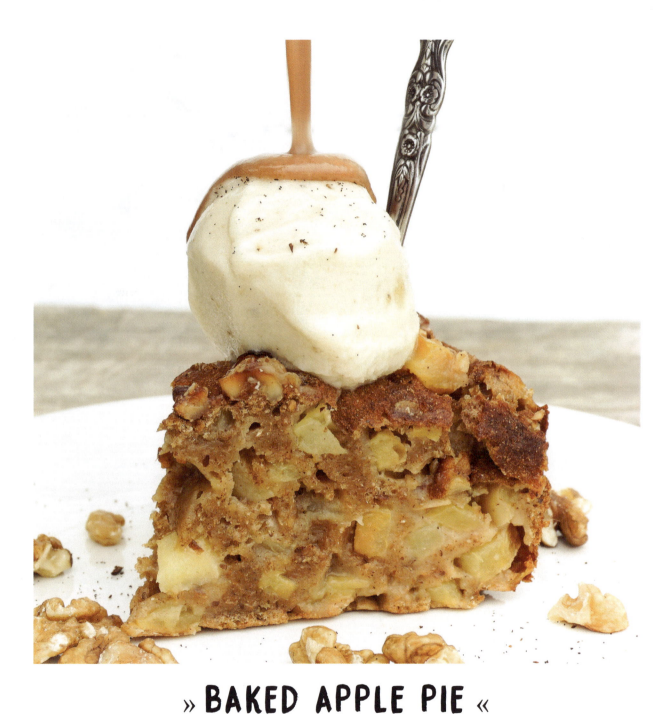

» BAKED APPLE PIE «

WITH VANILLA 'NICE CREAM' AND CARAMEL SAUCE

APPLE PIE

2 1/4 cups whole wheat flour

1 cup almond milk

1/4 cup orange juice

1/4 cup apple sauce

1/4 cup maple syrup

3 apples, diced

2 flax 'eggs' (2 Tbsp ground flax seeds + 4 Tbsp water)

1 Tbsp baking powder

1 tsp cinnamon & ginger

ICE CREAM

3 frozen bananas

A dash of almond milk

1 tsp ground vanilla bean

CARAMEL SAUCE

6 Medjool dates, pitted

1/3 cup coconut milk

1 tsp vanilla extract

Apple pies are a must-have in every dessert collection. Traditional apple pies are loaded with butter, eggs and saturated fats. This version, in contrast, is much healthier. The combination of warm apple pie with vanilla ice cream and sweet date caramel sauce is just perfect!

1. Preheat the oven to 200°C/400°F.

2. Place the diced apples, flour, baking powder & spices into a bowl and mix together.

3. Combine the remaining liquid ingredients in a bowl, whisk together and slowly add to the apple-flour mixture.

4. Use a spatula to combine the ingredients until you have a smooth batter.

5. Line a cake tin (8" or 20cm) with parchment paper, pour the cake batter inside and place in the oven for 45-50 minutes.

6. For both the vanilla ice cream and the caramel sauce, simply add all ingredients to a high-speed belnder and blend until smooth.

7. Serve the warm apple pie with a scoop of vanilla ice cream and caramel sauce on top!

> **TiP HOW TO MAKE HEALTHY ICE CREAM**
>
> Frozen bananas have the perfect texture to make a tasty ice cream. Simply place them in a blender with a dash of vegan milk and voilà!

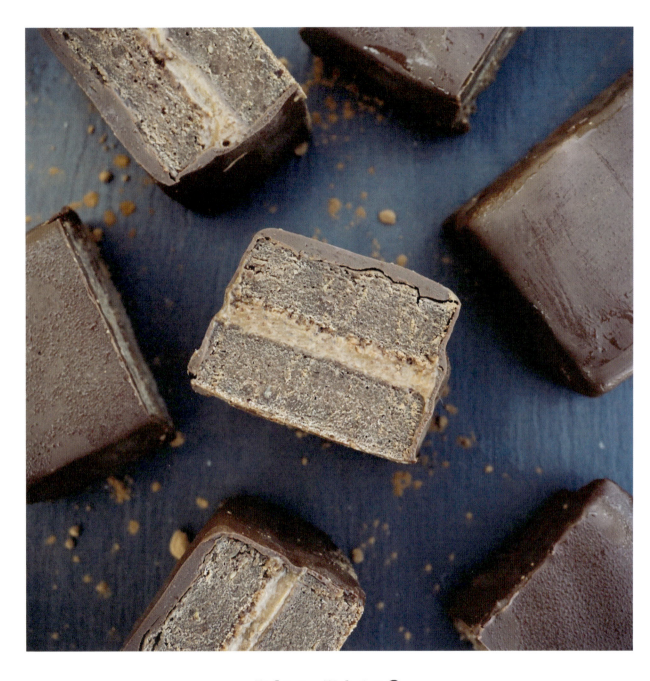

» TIM TAMS «

serves 8

BISCUIT

1 cup spelt flour

1/4 cup almond milk

1/8 cup apple sauce

1/3 cup maple syrup

1/4 cup full-fat coconut cream

1/3 cup cacao powder

1 flax 'egg'

1 tsp vanilla extract

FILLING

1 cup Medjool dates, pitted

1/4 cup coconut cream

1/4 cup cacao powder

1 tsp vanilla extract

COATING

1 bar dark vegan chocolate

Healthy vegan Tim Tams are here! Instead of tons of sugar and additives, these Tim Tams include only good ingredients and natural sweeteners to give you the same chocolaty experience - but healthier!

1. Preheat the oven to 175°C/350°F.
2. Sift the flour and cacao powder in a bowl and beat the remaining liquid ingredients in a separate bowl.
3. Combine dry and liquid ingredients beating on low speed and place the bowl in the freezer for 45 minutes.
4. Line a bread loaf tin or square tin with parchment paper and place half of the dough inside. 5. Bake for 12-15 minutes and repeat this step with the second half so that you have two equal biscuit parts.
6. In the meantime place all filling ingredients in a high-speed blender until smooth.
7. Once the biscuit has cooled down, spread the filling in between the two biscuit layers and place in the freezer. When firm, cut into squares and coat with melted dark vegan chocolate (I cut fairly big squares and cut them in half again).

NOTE

For this recipe I used a 8" (20cm) bread loaf tin.

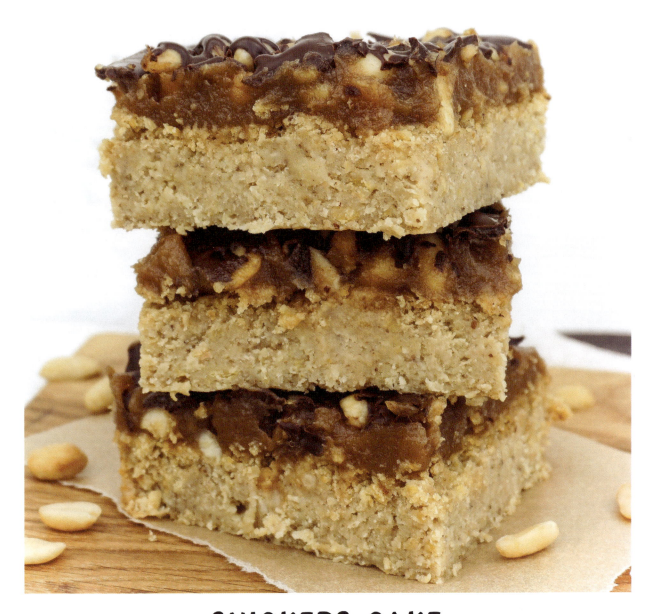

» SNICKERS CAKE «

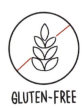

GLUTEN-FREE

CAKE

1 can chickpeas (14oz), drained and rinsed

1 cup oat flour

1/4 cup maple syrup

1/2 cup almond milk

1/3 cup natural peanut butter

1 tsp vanilla extract

1 tsp baking powder

1 Tbsp ground flax seeds

CARAMEL

12 Medjool dates, pitted

1/3 cup water

1/8 cup almond milk

1/2 tsp vanilla extract

1/8 tsp sea salt

TOPPINGS

1/3 cup unsalted peanuts, chopped

3-4 pieces dark vegan chocolate, melted

Snickers has always been my favorite chocolate bar. The combination of caramel, chocolate and peanuts is just unbeatable. This version is so much healthier and makes a delicious, naturally-sweetened cake to serve friends or family!

1. Preheat the oven to 175°C/350°C.

2. Place all cake ingredients in a high-speed blender until you get a smooth dough.

3. Line a square baking tin (8"x 8") with parchment paper and place the dough inside. Press down evenly and bake in the oven for 30-35 minutes.

4. In the meantime, make the caramel by simply blending up all ingredients until smooth.

5. Once the cake is done, let it cool down and spread the caramel on top.

6. Add the unsalted peanuts and slightly press them into the caramel. Place in the freezer while you melt the chocolate.

7. Drizzle the melted chocolate on top and place back into the freezer for 20 minutes.

TiP **HEALTH BENEFITS OF DATES**

Dates are nature's chewy caramel that is jam-packed with iron, calcium, potassium, magnesium and copper. Dates are rich in fiber, easily digestible and work wonders against constipation, free radicals and inflammation.

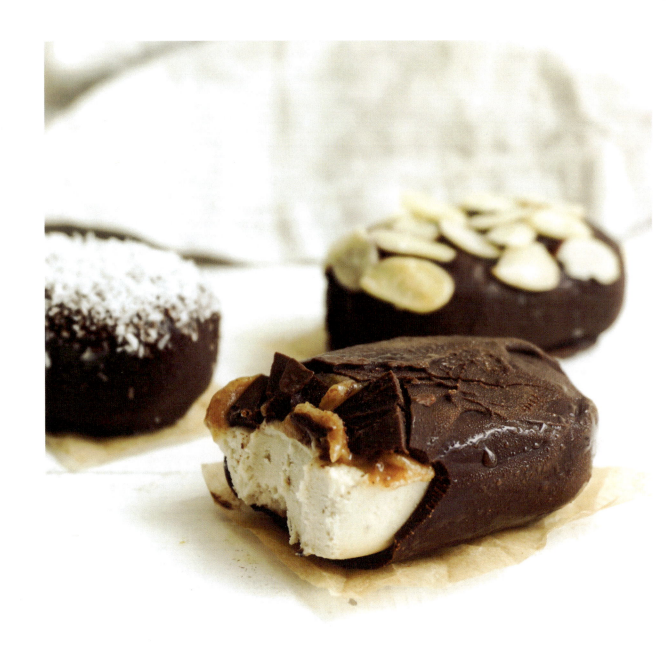

» CARAMEL FILLED MAGNUM «

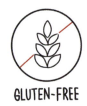

GLUTEN-FREE

serves 8

◇◇◇◇◇◇◇◇◇◇◇◇◇◇◇◇◇◇◇◇◇◇◇◇◇◇◇◇◇

ICE CREAM

1/2 cup cashews, soaked overnight

1/2 cup coconut cream

1 tsp ground vanilla bean

1/8 cup maple syrup

SALTED CARAMEL

6 Medjool dates, pitted

1/4 cup coconut cream

1/2 tsp ground vanilla bean

Pinch of sea salt

COATING

1 bar dark vegan chocolate,
melted

Healthy Magnums, say what?! A creamy ice cream filling, layered with ooey-gooey caramel, surrounded by a crunchy chocolate shell! Dairy-free, refined sugar-free and extremely tasty.

◇◇◇

1. Place all the ice cream ingredients into a blender and mix until smooth.

2. Pour the ice cream mixture into the molds until they are 3/4 full (don't fill them up completely so you have some space left for the caramel).

3. Add the wooden sticks and place the filled molds into the freezer for about 1 hour.

4. In the meantime place all caramel ingredients into the blender and mix them until you get a creamy texture (you will have to use your blender stick to mash up the dates). Spread the caramel evenly into the remaining ¼ of the molds.

5. Place the molds back into the freezer for 1-2 hours until the caramel has hardened up. Once firm, cover in melted chocolate and add desired toppings (nuts, coconut).

TIP
These ice cream molds can be found on www.thetastyk. com/equipment

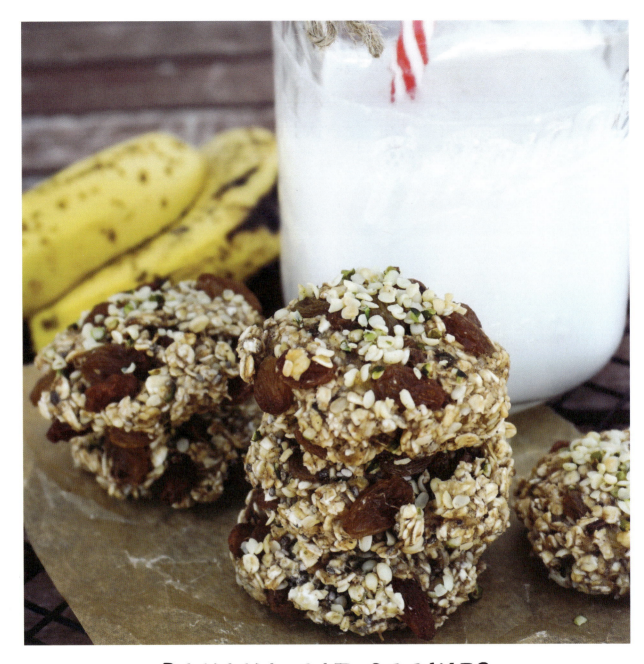

» BANANA OAT COOKIES «

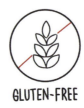

GLUTEN-FREE

serves 8

INGREDIENTS

1 cup rolled oats

2 ripe bananas

1/8 cup hemp seeds

1 tsp cinnamon

1/3 cup raisins (or dark vegan chocolate chips)

1 Tbsp flax seeds

1/2 tsp ground vanilla bean

TOPPINGS

Hemp seeds

Dessicated coconut

Looking for a super healthy and nutritious snack? Here you go! These super simple banana oat cookies are loaded with nutrients and healthy carbs to satisfy your sweet tooth. They take less than 15 minutes to make and store amazingly in an air-tight container to enjoy throughout the week!

1. Preheat the oven to 175°C/350°F.
2. Place the bananas in a bowl and mash them up with a fork.
3. Add the remaining ingredients and combine with a spatula.
4. Line a baking tin with parchment paper and small form cookies with your hands (at this point you can add desired toppings).
5. Place them on the sheet and bake for 10-15 minutes.
6. Let the cookies cool down and enjoy!

TiP HEALTH BENEFITS OF HEMP SEEDS

Hemp seeds work wonders for improving digestion, metabolism and balance hormones. They contain a perfect 3:1 ratio of omega-3 and omega-6 fatty acids, which promotes cardivascular health and also contain all 20 amino acids.

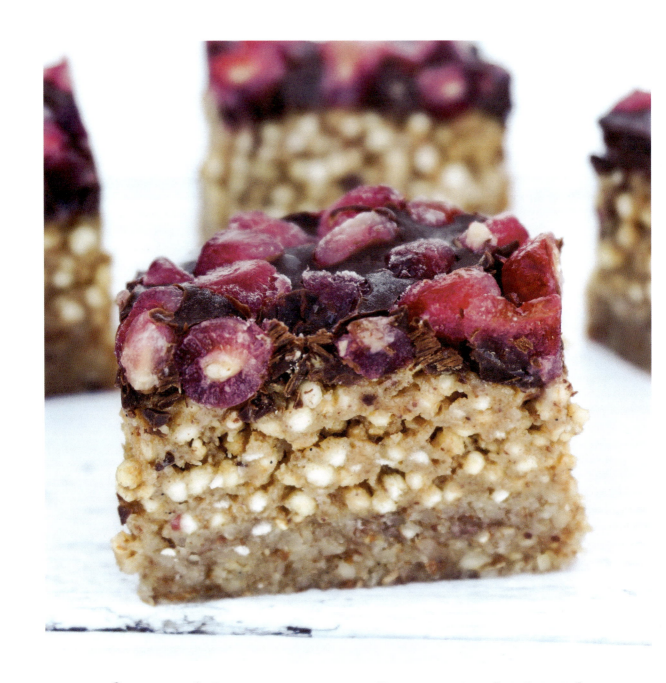

» POMEGRANATE CARAMEL SLICES «

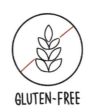

GLUTEN-FREE

serves 14-16

CRUST

1 cup raw almonds

1/4 cup rolled oats

6 Medjool dates, pitted

2-3 Tbsp almond milk

1 tsp vanilla extract

CARAMEL LAYER

12 Medjool dates, pitted

1/8 cup almond milk

1 cup raw buckwheat or puffed quinoa

1 Tbsp almond butter

1/8 tsp sea salt

1/3 cup water

TOPPINGS

1 bar dark vegan chocolate, melted

1 cup pomegranate seeds

Pomegranate, chocolate and caramel - could this combination get any better? These crispy caramel slices are dreamy pieces of fruit & crunchy. The perfect treat to store in the freezer and enjoy ice cold! Naturally sweetened with ooey-gooey dates, gluten-free and oh so yummy!

1. Place all the crust ingredients in a high-speed blender and mix until combined.

2. Line a square baking tin with parchment paper, press the crust down evenly and place in the freezer to firm up.

3. For the caramel layer, place the dates, almond milk, water, almond butter and salt in the blender until you get a smooth mixture. Add the date mixture into a bowl and stir in the buckwheat/ quinoa.

4. Spread the caramel layer on top of the crust and place it back into the freezer.

5. Melt the chocolate and pour over the carmel layer. Immediately sprinkle the pomegranate seeds on top and freeze for another 15 minutes.

NOTE
For this recipe I used a 8" x 8" (20cm x 20cm) square cake tin.

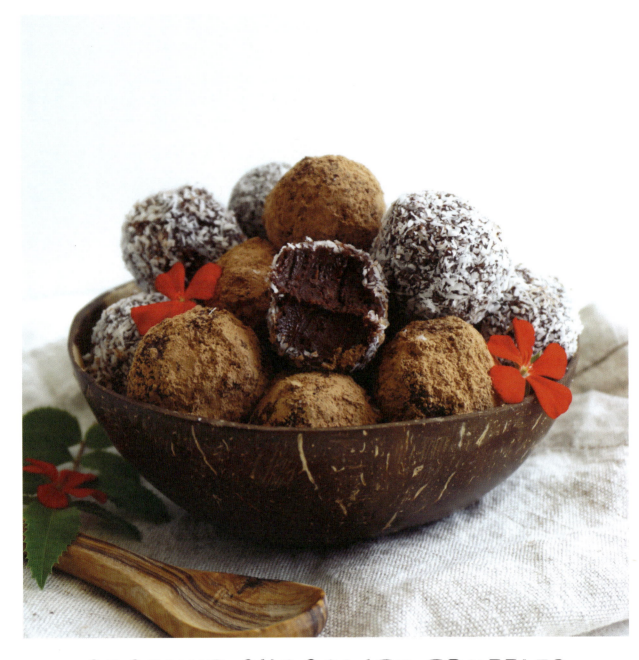

» COCONUT CHOCOLATE TRUFFLES «

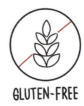

GLUTEN-FREE

serves 12

INGREDIENTS

150gr dark vegan chocolate

1/2 cup full fat coconut cream

1/4 cup desiccated coconut (+ more for rolling)

1/2 tsp vanilla extract

TOPPINGS

Nuts

Oats

Raw cacao powder

These amazing coconut chocolate truffles are just heavenly. They are by far one of the easiest treats to make and literally melt in your mouth! All you need is 4 basic ingredients and that's it. You can always extend the basic version and add in some other exciting stuff, but for me, in this case, less is more!

1. Break the chocolate into pieces and melt it (I just put it into a glass bowl and place it into a sauce pan filled with boiling water).

2. Once the chocolate is completely melted, add the coconut cream and stir until smooth.

3. Add the vanilla extract and the shredded coconut and mix well until combined.

4. Place the bowl into the freezer and let chill for 30 minutes.

5. Take it out from the freezer and form small balls with you hands. This is going to be a bit messy but it's worth it! If you want add one walnut/ almond inside and roll the truffle in shredded coconut/ oats/ cacao powder/ granola.

6. Put the truffles back into the fridge until the firm up or eat them immediately!

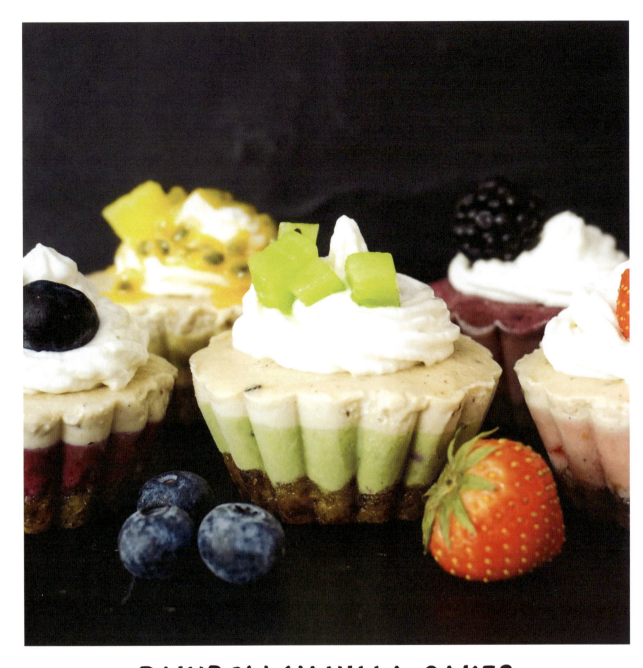

» RAINBOW VANILLA CAKES «

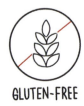

GLUTEN-FREE

serves 10

CRUST

1/2 cup walnuts

10 Medjool dates, pitted

1/2 tsp ground vanilla bean

FILLING

1/2 cup cashews, soaked overnight

1/2 cup coconut cream

1/4 cup maple syrup

1 tsp ground vanilla bean

• • • • •

1/8 cup strawberries
1/8 cup blueberries
1/8 cup kiwi
1/8 cup pineapple

TOPPING

Coconut whipped cream (see p.15)

These cute rainbow vanilla cakes are the perfect dessert to impress friends! They're super easy to make and taste deliciously creamy with a fruity touch. Combine your favorite fruits and make colorful cakes for any kind of celebration!

1. Place the crust ingredients in a high-speed blender/food processor and blend.

2. Divide the crust into 10 equal parts, press down evenly into silicone muffin cups and place in the freezer.

3. Place the base filling ingredients in the blender and mix until smooth. Pour half of the mixture in a glass and set aside.

4. Divide the other half into 4 parts, add one fresh fruit to each and blend until smooth.

5. Pour the fruit mixtures on top of the crusts until half of the muffin cups are filled and place in the freezer to set.

6. Once firm, add the vanilla mixture as a second laer and return to the freezer.

7. Top with coconut whipped cream and fresh fruit pieces!

TiP
Dates have the perfect texture and natural sweetness to make raw cake crust. Opt for Medjool dates, as they are super gooey and sweet.

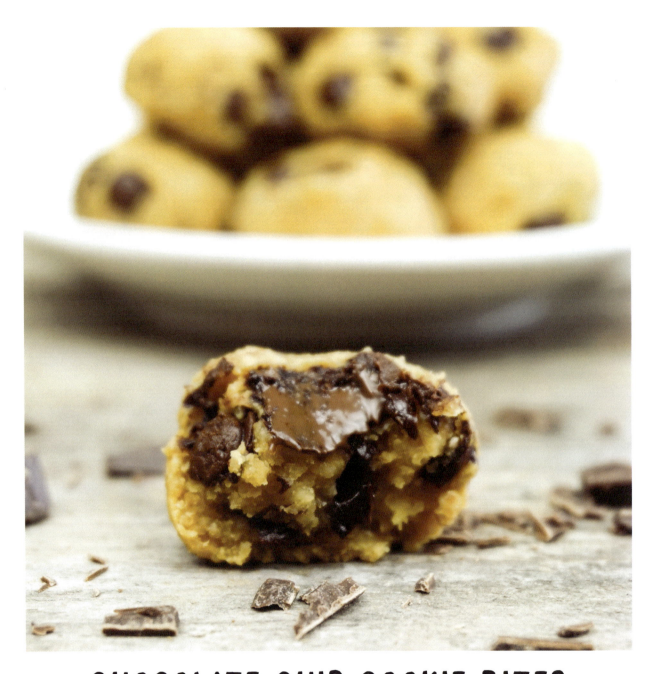

» CHOCOLATE CHIP COOKIE BITES «

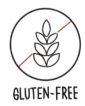

GLUTEN-FREE

serves 20

~~~~~~~~~~~~~~~~~~~~~~~~~~~~~~~~~~

INGREDIENTS

1 can chickpeas (15oz), drained
and rinsed

1/3 cup oat flour

1/4 cup natural peanut butter,
melted

1/8 cup almond milk

1/4 cup maple syrup

1/2 tsp vanilla extract

1 tsp baking powder

• • • • •

1/3 cup dark vegan chocolate
chips

Healthy Chocolate Chip Cookie Bites? Yes, it is possible! Believe me, you won't be wanting any other cookies after you've tried these. Jam-packed with protein, these little bundles of joy have a soft core with melted chocolate and are slightly crunchy on the outside – so good!

~~~~~~

1. Preheat the oven to 175°C/350°F and line a baking tray with parchment paper.

2. Place the first 7 ingredients in your high-speed blender/ food processor and use the blender stick to mash them down until you have a more or less smooth batter.

3. Place the batter in a bowl, add in the chocolate chips and combine with a spatula.

4. Use your hands to form small bite-sized balls and place on the baking tray.

5. Place the tray in the oven and bake for 10-15 minutes.

TIP **HEALTH BENEFITS OF CHICKPEAS**

Chickpeas, like other legumes, are extremely high in protein and fiber, and also contain numerous vitamins and minerals. They effectively lower blood sugar levels and cholestorol.

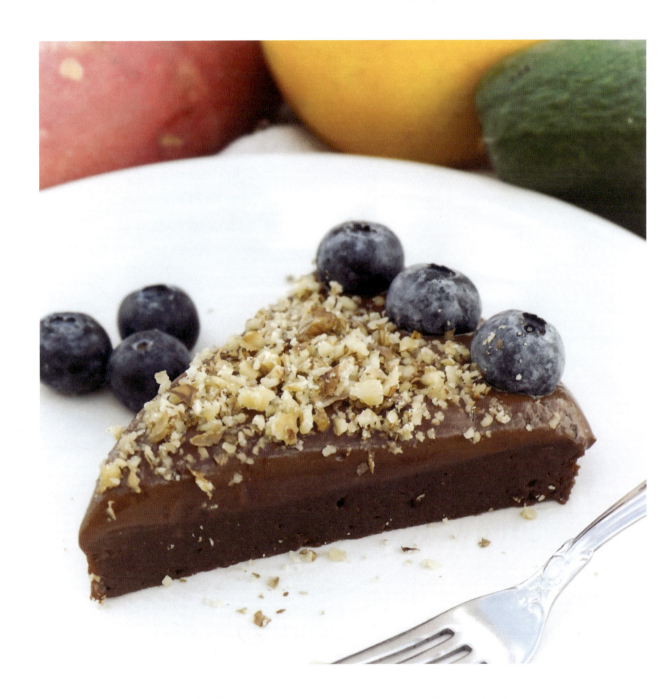

» VEGGIE CHOCOLATE TART «

Serves 10

TART

1 small zucchini, leave the skin on

1 cup baby spinach

1 small sweet potato, cooked

1 1/2 cups spelt flour

1/3 cup full-fat coconut cream

1/2 cup cacao powder

8 Medjool dates, pitted

4 Tbsp maple syrup

1 tsp baking powder

1 flax egg

FROSTING

1 ripe avocado

1/4 cup maple syrup

1/4 cup cacao powder

1/3 cup coconut cream

1/2 tsp vanilla extract

Vegetables in desserts? Don't judge until you've tried it! Chocolaty desserts are especially perfect to sneak in greens, beans and veggies, as the strong chocolate taste will completely take over your taste buds. Like this, you get a fudgy chocolate tart full of nutrients with a super sweet and creamy avocado frosting!

1. Preheat the oven to 175°C/350°F.

2. Place all the tart ingredients into a high-speed blender and blend for 1 minute until you have a smooth batter.

3. Grease a baking tin with coconut oil and pour the batter inside.

4. Place in the oven and bake for 10-15 minutes.

5. In the meantime make the frosting. Place all the ingredients into your blender and mix until smooth.

6. Let the tart cool down before spreading the frosting on top. Add berries and crushed nuts as toppings and enjoy!

TIP HEALTH BENEFITS OF AVOCADOS

Avocados are incredibly nutritious fruits. They are loaded with heart-healthy monounsaturated fatty acids, fiber and contain more potassium than bananas. Those healthy fats help absorb the nutrients from plant foods.

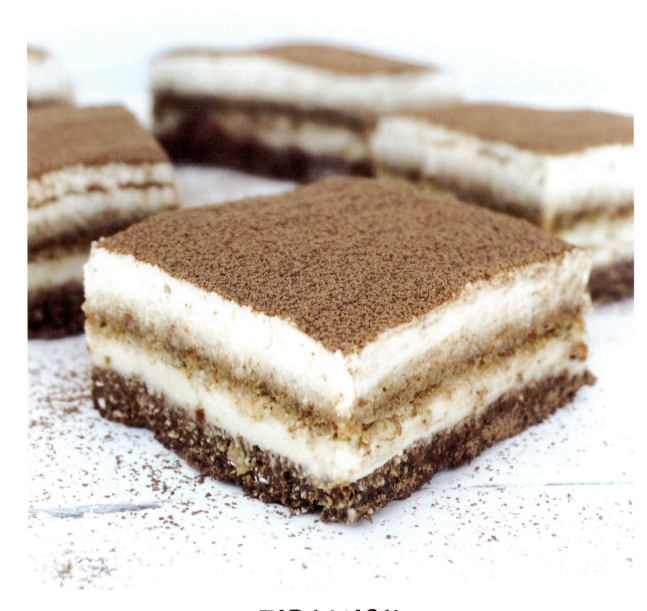

» TIRAMISU «

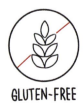

GLUTEN-FREE

serves 8-10

CRUST

1.5 cups rolled oats

1 cup Medjool dates, pitted

4 Tbsp cold espresso

1/2 tsp vanilla extract

2 Tbsp cacao powder

LADYFINGERS

1 cup almond meal

2 Tbsp coconut flour

6 Medjool dates, pitted

3 Tbsp cold espresso

1 tsp vanilla extract

VANILLA CREAM

2 cups cashews, soaked

1/3 cup coconut cream (only the firm part)

1/8 cup maple syrup

1 tsp vanilla extract

1.5 cups water, as needed

Everybody loves tiramisu! While traditional tiramisu is extremely heavy and loaded with cream and sugar, this version is much healthier, refined sugar-free and made with only wholesome ingredients. You'll enjoy every bite of this deliciousness!

1. For the crust, place the oats into your high-speed blender and pulse until you have flour. Add the remaining ingredients until you have a sticky dough.

2. Press evenly into the bottom of a lined square baking tin and set in the fridge.

3. For the ladyfinger, follow the same instructions (first oats, then remaining ingredients). Form into rectangular cookies that will fit into the baking pan.

4. For the vanilla cream, add all ingredients into your blender until you reach a smooth, pudding-like consistency, adding water as needed.

5. Spread half the cream on the crust, place the ladyfingers close beside each other on top and add the rest of the cream.

6. Set in the fridge or freezer for at least 24 hours. Dust with cacao powder and slice with a sharp knife before serving.

NOTE
For this recipe I used a 8" x 8" (20cm x 20cm) square cake tin.

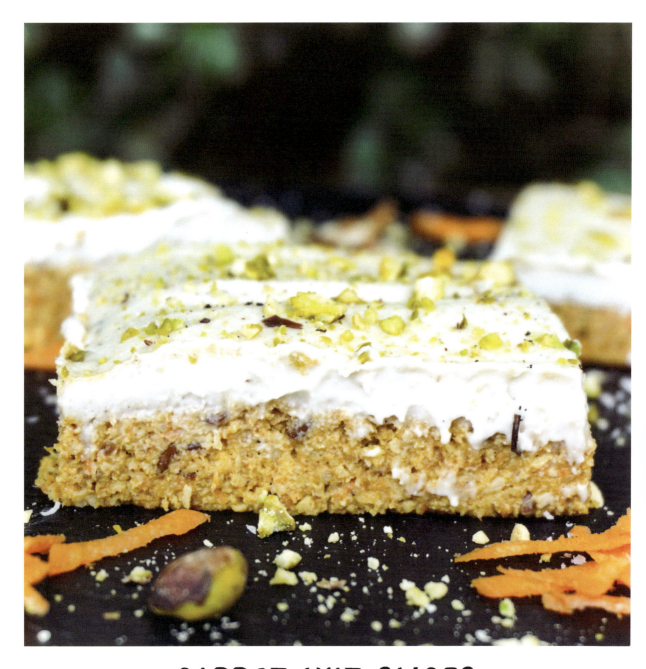

» CARROT NUT SLICES «

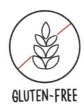

GLUTEN-FREE

serves 10-12

BASE

1.5 cups carrots, grated

1 cup walnuts

1 cup Medjool dates, pitted

1/2 cup shredded coconut

1/3 cup oats

1 tsp vanilla extract

1 Tbsp flaxseeds

1 tsp cinnamon

1/4 tsp ground ginger & nutmeg

FROSTING

1 cup cashews, soaked

1/3 cup coconut cream

3 Tbsp maple syrup

1/2 tsp vanilla bean powder

1 Tbsp fresh lemon juice

These delicious carrot nut slices are a raw version of the classic baked carrot cake. Refined sugar-free, gluten-free and topped with creamy cashew frosting, they are the perfect healthy treat for every occasion!

1. For the dough, place all the base ingredients in a high-speed blender until combined (if it's too mushy add more oats or shredded coconut).

2. Line a baking tray with parchment paper and place the dough inside. Use a spatula to evenly press the dough down. Place in the freezer while you make the frosting.

3. Place all the ingredients for the frosting into your high-speed blender and mix until smooth. Once creamy, pour it over the hardened dough and spread evenly.

4. Top with crushed pistachios, more ground vanilla beans and place in the fridge or freezer (make sure to let it cool down at room temperature before eating).

> **TiP BENEFITS OF SOAKING NUTS**
>
> Soaking nuts helps to absorb mineral and vitamins by removing enzymes calles phytates. Since nuts have a high amount of enzymes inhibitors, soaking neutralizes the enzymes and allows for proper digestion.

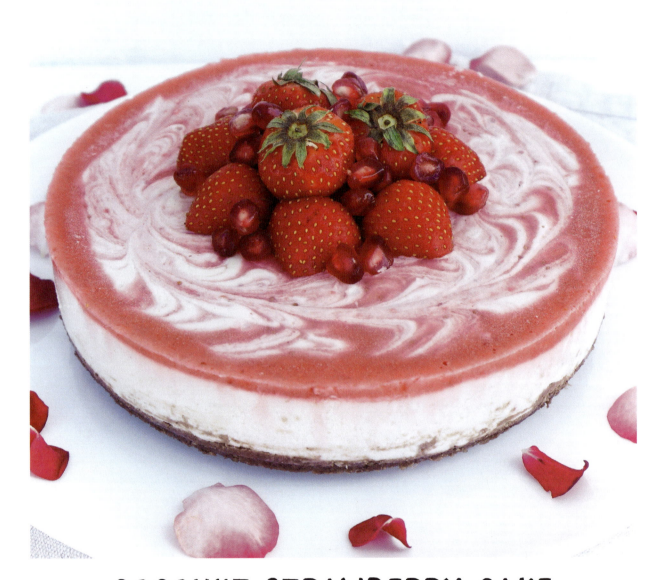

» COCONUT STRAWBERRY CAKE «

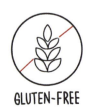

GLUTEN-FREE

◇◇◇◇◇◇◇◇◇◇◇◇◇◇◇◇◇◇◇◇◇◇◇◇◇◇◇◇◇◇◇◇

CRUST

10 Medjool dates, pitted

1/2 cup almonds

1/3 cup desiccated coconut

1/8 cup cacao powder

1 tsp ground vanilla bean

1 Tbsp water

CREAM FILLING

2 cups cashews, soaked

1 cup coconut cream

1/3 cup maple syrup

1 tsp vanilla extract

1/8 cup lemon juice

TOP LAYER

4 fresh straberries

1 Tbsp coconut milk

1 tsp lemon juice

This creamy coconut strawberry cake is the perfect treat for warm summer days. Fruity raw cakes are one of my favorites because they get most of their sweetness from fresh ripe fruits. Also they are amazingly pretty, easy to make and perfect to impress friends & family on any occasion!

◇◇◇◇◇◇◇◇◇◇◇◇◇◇◇◇◇◇◇◇◇◇◇◇◇◇◇◇◇◇◇◇

1. For the crust, place all ingredients into your high-speed blender and mix until you have a smooth dough.

2. Line a cake tin with parchment paper and press the dough down evely with your hands. Place in the freezer to set.

3. Prepare the cream filling by adding all ingredients into your blender. Mix until smooth.

4. Pour the cream filling over the crust and place back into the freezer.

5. Prepare the strawberry layer by blending all ingredients until smooth. Pour the layer over the cream filling and use a toothpick to create swirls (don't overdo it). Top with your favorite berries, chocolate and nuts.

6. Place the cake back into the freezer until firm (2-3 hours). Before serving, let defrost at room temperature and enjoy!

NOTE
For this recipe I used a 8" (20cm) round cake tin.

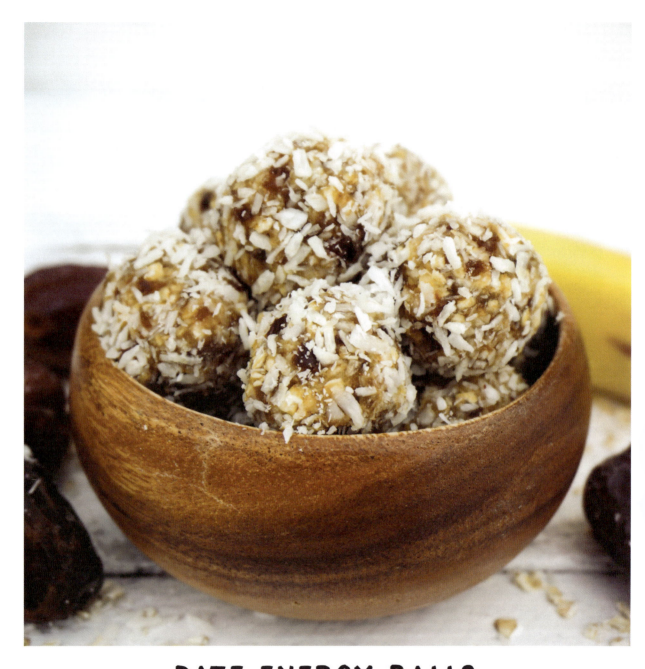

» DATE ENERGY BALLS «

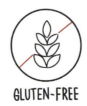

GLUTEN-FREE

serves 10

INGREDIENTS

1 ripe banana

6 Medjool dates, pitted

1/4 cup desiccated coconut

3/4 cup rolled oats

1/3 cup walnuts

1 Tbsp chia seeds

COATING

Desiccated coconut

Oats

Chia seeds

These little energy balls are a great way to make use of ooey-gooey dates. They are a perfect treat and go-to when you're craving something sweet but want to keep your efforts to a minimum. I always make sure to have them on hand and like to experiment with many variations of these delicious energy balls!

1. Place the oats, desiccated coconut, walnuts and chia seeds in your high-speed blender and pulse until crumbly.

2. Add the dates and banana and blend. Use your blender stick to mash down the ingredients until you get a more or less smooth mixture (I prefer having some whole pieces inside). You want the mixture to be a bit sticky but not too much so that you can still handle it easily.

3. Use your hands to form small bite-sized balls and coat with more coconut, oats or chia seeds.

4. Store in the fridge and enjoy!

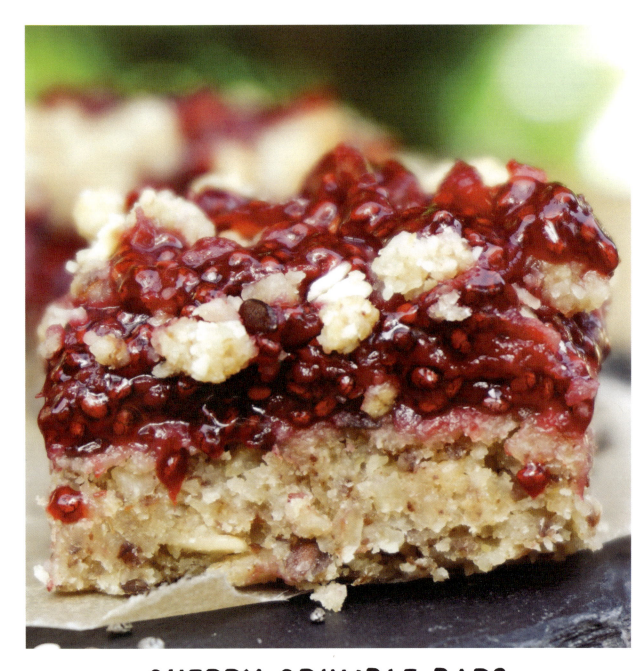

» CHERRY CRUMBLE BARS «

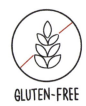

GLUTEN-FREE

BASE

1 cup oat flour

1 cup almond flour (make your own by blending almonds)

2 flax 'eggs' (2 Tbsp ground flax seeds + 4 Tbsp water)

2 Tbsp almond butter

1/8 cup almond milk

1/8 cup maple syrup

1 tsp baking powder

1/8 tsp sea salt

CHIA JAM

300gr frozen cherries

5 Tbsp chia seeds

1 Tbsp lemon juice

1 tsp vanilla extract

3 Tbsp maple syrup

These delicious cherry crumble bars are super light and loaded with fresh summery flavors. You can easily change the cherries to any other fruit of your choice which makes this treat super versatile and extremely tasty!

1. For the chia jam, heat up a sauce pan, cook the cherries until soft and add the remaning ingredients. Mash the cherries with a fork until smooth and let cool down in the fridge for 2 hours.

2. Prepare the flax 'eggs' and set aside for 5-10 minutes. Preheat the oven to 175°C/350°F.

3. Mix up all base ingredients in a medium sized bowl and combine. Take out 1/4 of the crumble dough and set aside.

4. Line a brownie tin with parchment paper and place the remaining 3/4 of the dough inside. Spread evenly and bake for 10 minutes.

5. Take it out of the oven and spread the cherry chia jam evenly on top. Crumble up the remaining 1/4 of dough and sprinkle it on top of the jam layer.

6. Place the tin back into the oven and bake at the same temperature for another 20 minutes. Let cool down before cutting!

NOTE

For this recipe I used a 8" x 8" (20cm x 20cm) square cake tin.

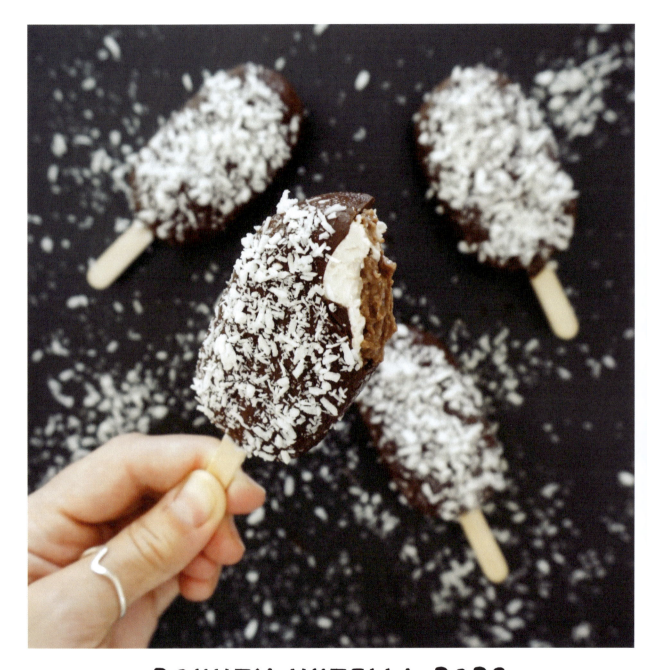

» BOUNTY NUTELLA POPS «

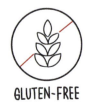

GLUTEN-FREE

COCO FILLING

1/4 cup cashews, soaked

1/3 cup coconut cream

1/2 tsp ground vanilla bean

2 Tbsp maple syrup

1/4 cup desiccated coconut

NUTELLA

1 cup roasted hazelnuts

1/4 cup cacao powder

1/4 cup coconut cream

1/4 cup maple syrup

1 tsp vanilla extract

1/8 tsp sea salt

COATING

200 gr dark vegan chocolate

Desiccated coconut

Bounty Nutella ice cream? Three of my favourite things combined in one treat! A smooth Nutella core, surrounded by creamy coconut ice cream, coated with crispy dark chocolate. Sounds like a winner to me!

1. For the coconut filling, simply place all ingredients into a high-speed blender and mix until smooth.

2. Pour the coconut filling into your ice cream molds until they are half full and place them into the freezer for 30 minutes.

3. Prepare the nutella by simply blending the hazelnuts until crumbly, and then adding all other ingredients. Blend everything together until smooth.

4. Take out the molds, spread a thin nutella layer on top of the first coconut layer and place back into the freezer for 15 minutes.

5. Pour the remaning coconut filling on top of the nutella layer and let set in the fridge.

6. Once firm, cover with melted dark chocolate and sprinkle desiccated coconut on top. Let defrost for a while before eating!

TiP
These ice cream molds can be found on www.thetastyk.com/equipment

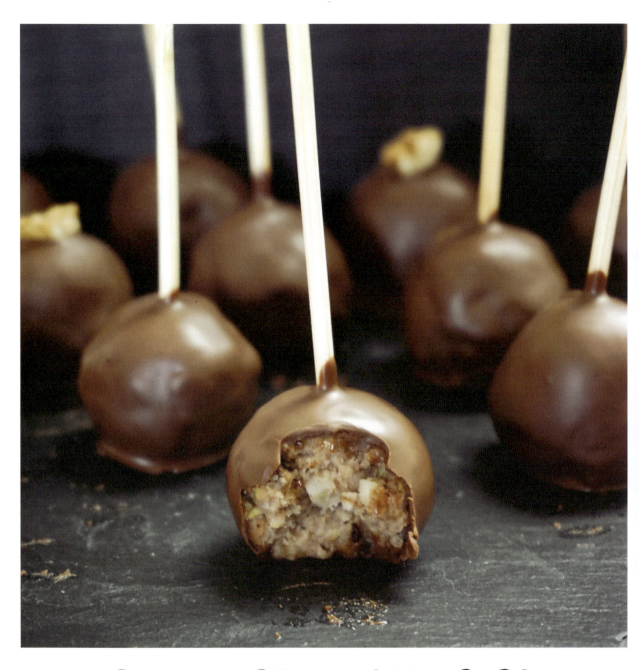

» BANANA BREAD CAKE POPS «

serves 8-10

BANANA BREAD

1 ripe banana

1/2 cup almond milk

1/2 cup oat flour

1/4 cup whole wheat flour

1 tsp chia seeds

1 tsp ground flax seeds

1 tsp date syrup

1/2 tsp baking powder

1/4 tsp vanilla extract

1/4 tsp cinnamon

1/8 cup walnuts, chopped

COATING

200 gr dark vegan chocolate

These delicious banana bread cake pops are the perfect twist of the classic dessert (or breakfast)! Soft banana bread dough, filled with crunchy walnuts and coated with a yummy chocolate shell – could it get any better than this?

1. Preheat the oven to 175°C/350°F and grease a small cake tin with coconut oil.

2. For the banana bread, place the ripe banana into a bowl and mash it with a fork.

3. Add the remaining ingredients to the bowl and whisk together.

4. Pour the batter into the cake tin and bake in the oven for about 20 minutes (until toothpick comes out clean).

5. Let the cake cool down for 5-10 minutes and start breaking it apart. Take a small portion of the bread and roll it in your hands to form little balls.

6. Once you have rolled the whole bread into balls, place a skewer into each ball.

7. Melt your vegan dark chocolate and dip each ball into the chocolate. Place in the freezer/fridge until firm and enjoy!

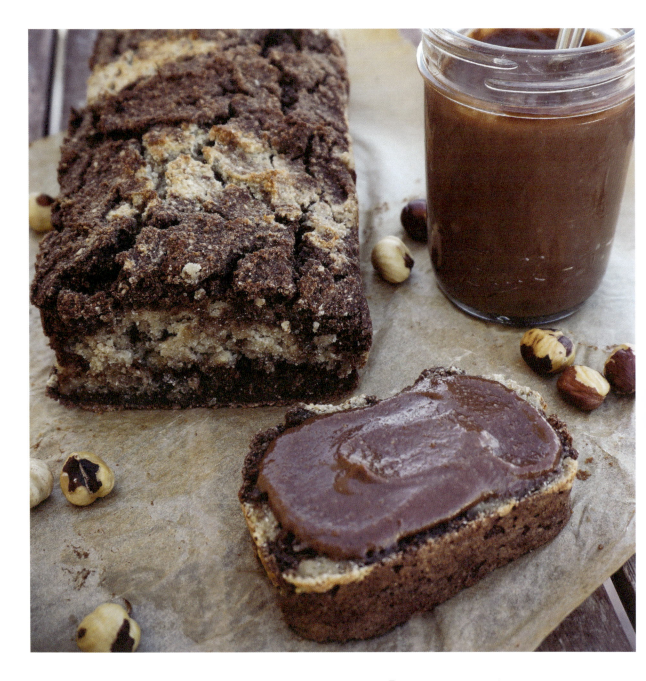

» CHOCOLATE MARBLE CAKE «

serves 8

CAKE

3 cups oat flour

1 cup spelt flour

3 ripe bananas

3/4 cup rice milk

1 tsp vanilla extract

1 Tbsp ground flaxseeds

1/3 cup + 2 Tbsp maple syrup

1/3 cup cacao powder

1 Tbsp baking powder

TOPPINGS

Healthy Nutella (see p.57)

Dark vegan chocolate

While traditional marble cakes are loaded with refined sugars, oil and saturated fats, this cake is a much healthier version of the classic. Top with creamy Nutella or a chocolate coating for an extra twist and get hooked at the first bite!

1. Place the flour, flaxseeds and baking powder in a bowl and mix.

2. Place the bananas, rice milk, 1/3 cup of maple syrup and vanilla in a blender and combine.

3. Gently fold the liquid ingredients into the dry and use a spatula to combine.

4. Separate the batter into two equal parts. Into one part, add the cacao powder and 2 Tbsp of maple syrup and mix together.

5. Preheat the oven to 175°C/350°F.

6. Line a bread loaf tin with parchment paper. Scoop one big spoon of each batter after another into the tin until all gone.

7. Use a toothpick to create swirl patterns and place in the oven for 40-45 minutes (until toothpick comes out clean). Let cool down for 30 minutes before cutting.

8. Enjoy with Nutella (see p. 57) or melted dark vegan chocolate on top.

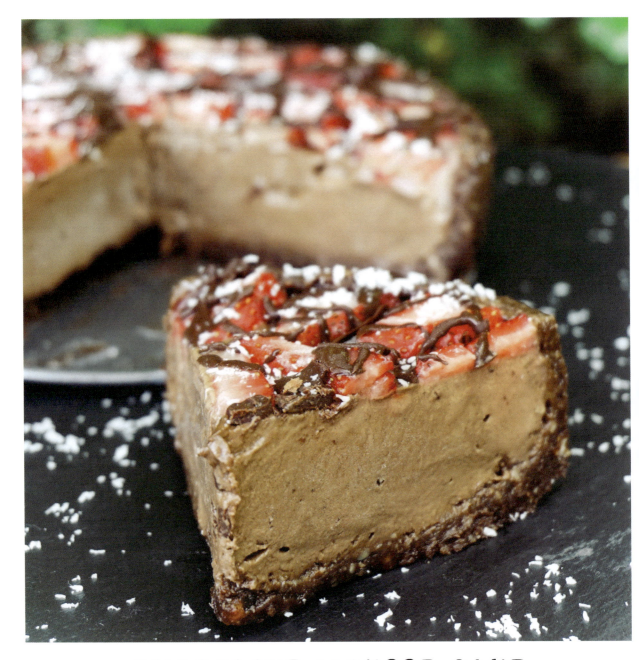

» CHOCOLATE MOUSSE CAKE «

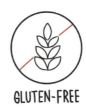

GLUTEN-FREE

CRUST

1/2 cup desiccated coconut

1/2 cup walnuts

1/4 cup almonds

12 Medjool dates, pitted

2 Tbsp cacao powder

FILLING

3/4 cup full-fat coconut cream

1/4 cup cacao powder

1/3 cup date syrup

1 ripe avocado

1 ripe banana

2 Tbsp almond butter

4 pieces vegan dark chocolate, melted

TOPPINGS

Strawberries

Vegan dark chocolate, melted

This chocolate mousse cake is super creamy and extremely rich in taste! The combination of avocado, coconut cream and almond butter makes this delicious cake not only really nutritious but also gives it an amazing mousse texture! The perfect treat for birthdays, celebrations or to surprise your friends and family!

1. Place the nuts in a blender and pulse until ground. Add the remaining crust ingredients and blend until combined.

2. Line a cake tin with parchment paper. Add the crust dough to the tin and evenly press it down with your hands. Make sure to also press the dough about 2-3 cm up the sides. When done place into the freezer to set.

3. In the meantime, add all the ingredients for the filling into a blender and mix until combined. Pour the filling into the cake tin and place into the freezer for at least 4 hours.

4. Top the cake with your favourite fresh fruits and melted dark chocolate. Store in the freezer and let it soften at room temperature before eating!

> ### TiP
> Avocados are not only extremely nutritious but, thanks to its texture can be used as healthy alternatives to create delicious mousse and cakes. Don't worry, you won't taste a thing!

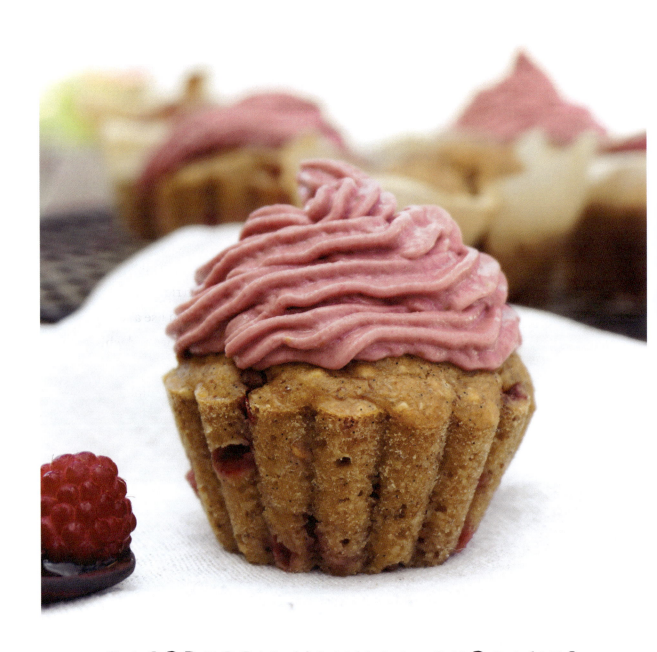

» RASPBERRY VANILLA CUPCAKES «

xxxxxxxxxxxxxxxxxxxxxxxxxxxxxxxxxx

CUPCAKES

1 cup oat flour

1 cup spelt flour

1 flax egg (1 Tbsp ground flax-
seed + 2 Tbsp water)

1 cup rice milk

1/8 cup apple sauce

1 ripe banana, mashed

1/4 cup maple syrup

1 Tbsp baking powder

1 tsp vanilla extract

1 1/2 cup frozen raspberries

FROSTING

1 can coconut cream (the firm
part)

1 Tbsp cup maple syrup

1/2 tsp vanilla extract

1/4 cup raspberries, mashed

Cupcakes are everyone's guilty pleasure. Not with these delicious fruity bites though. Refined sugar-free, oil-free and topped with a creamy coconut raspberry frosting, these little cakes will leave you wanting more!

xxxxxxxxxxxxxxxxxxxxxxxxxxxxxxxxxxxxxxxxxxx

1. Preheat the oven to 175°C/350°F.

2. Combine the dry ingredients in one bowl and the wet in another (except for the raspberries) and mix. Pour the wet ingredients into the dry and use a spatula to combine. Lastly add in the raspberries and whisk them under.

3. Spoon the batter into your cupcake molds (I use silicone ones) and place in the oven for 25-30 minutes (until toothpick comes out clean).

4. In the meantime, prepare the frosting. Place all the ingredients into a chilled bowl and whisk together until smooth. Add the frosting into a pipping bag and place in the freezer to firm up.

5. Let the cupcakes cool down and place the frosting on top!

TiP

The firm part of coconut cream serves as an excellent replacement for cream cheese in frostings of traditional recipes!

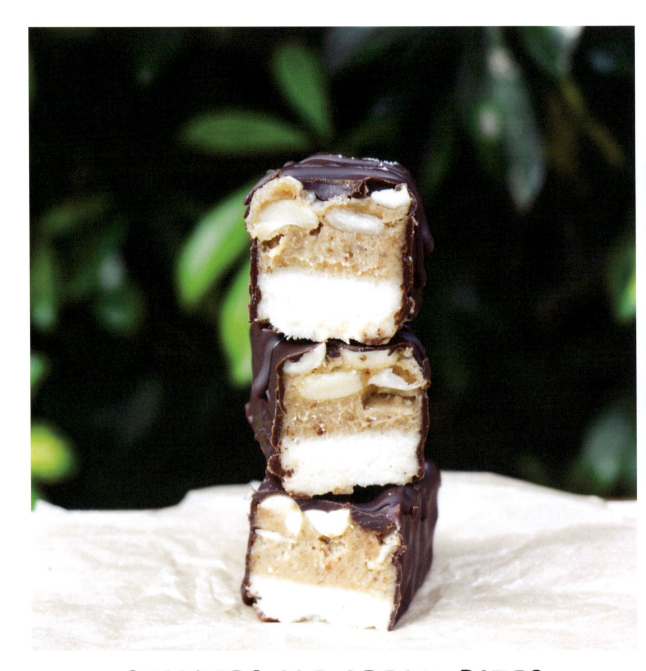

» SNICKERS ICE CREAM BITES «

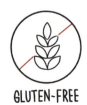

GLUTEN-FREE

serves 15

◇◇◇◇◇◇◇◇◇◇◇◇◇◇◇◇◇◇◇◇◇◇◇◇◇

NOUGAT

1 cup cashews, soaked overnight

2/3 cup full-fat coconut cream

2 Tbsp maple syrup

1/2 tsp vanilla extract

2/3 cup almond flour

CARAMEL

2 cups Medjool dates, pitted

1/2 cup natural peanut butter

3/4 cup coconut milk

1/4 tsp sea salt

1 1/2 cups unsalted peanuts,
roughly chopped

COATING

300gr vegan dark chocolate,
melted

If you are a fan of peanuts and chocolate, you will love these! These delicious snickers ice cream bites have been a huge success at many parties and gatherings so far. As a healthier but equally tasty alternative to the original they will leave you speechless!

◇◇◇◇◇◇◇◇◇◇◇◇◇◇◇◇◇◇◇◇◇◇◇◇◇◇◇◇◇◇◇◇◇◇◇

1. Place all the ingredients for the nougat layer (except for the almond flour) in a high speed blender or food processor and blend until smooth. Then add the almond flour and mix until combined.

2. Line a baking tin (8" x 8") with parchment paper and place the nougat layer inside. Spread the layer evenly and freeze for 2 hours.

3. In the meantime, place all the caramel ingredients (except for the peanuts) in a blender and mix until you get a smooth layer. When the nougat is firm, spread ½ of the caramel layer on top.

4. Sprinkle half of the chopped peanuts over the caramel layer and use a spatula to press the peanut pieces into the caramel. Repeat this step with the remaining caramel and peanuts and freeze for 1 hour.

5. Cut into desired shape (snickers bars size) and coat with melted dark chocolate. Store in the freezer, let dry and enjoy!

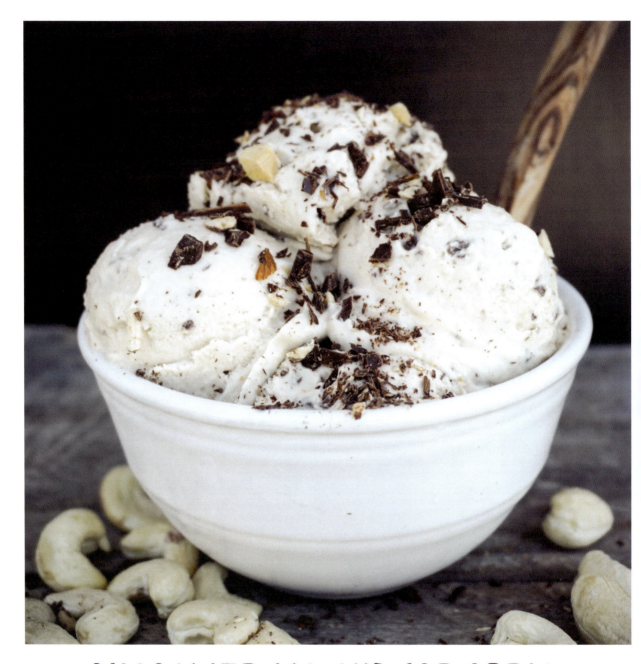

» CHOCOLATE ALMOND ICE CREAM «

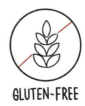

GLUTEN-FREE

serves 6-8

ICE CREAM

1 cup cashews, soaked overnight

1 14 oz can coconut cream

1/4 cup maple syrup

1 tsp vanilla extract

1/8 tsp sea salt

FILLING

1/2 bar dark vegan chocolate,
chopped into pieces

1/3 cup roasted almonds,
chopped into pieces

Who doesn't love ice cream - especially during summer?! This delicious and creamy chocolate almond ice cream hits all the right spots for the perfect treat! Best thing - you can make it without an ice cream maker!

1. Place all the ice cream ingredients into your high-speed blender and mix for 2-3 minutes until really smooth.

2. Pour the ice cream mixture into silicone trays (I use cupcake or ice cube trays) and place into the freezer overnight.

3. Once frozen, pop the ice cream out of the molds/ trays and place them into your blender. You might have to wait and let them defrost a bit. Blend again for 1-2 minutes and use your blender stick to mash down the mixture.

4. Once smooth, scoop the ice cream into a plastic box/ bowl, add in the copped chocolate and roasted almond pieces and combine.

5. Place back into the freezer for 1 hour and scoop out to serve.

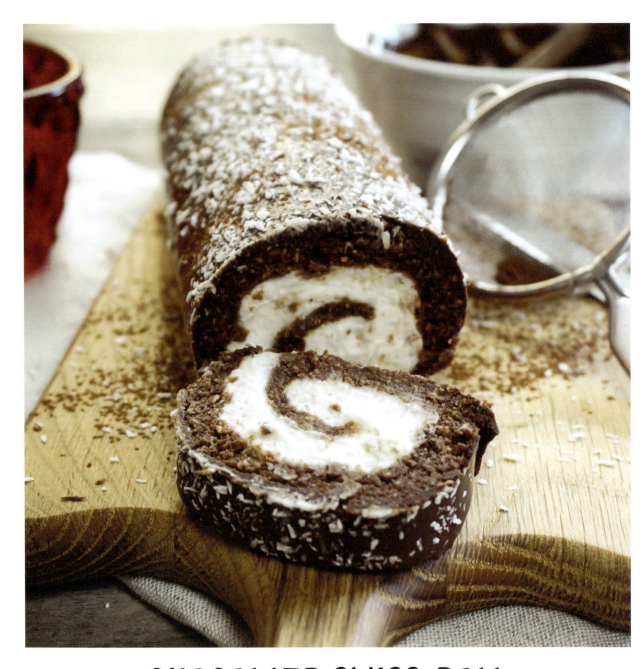

» CHOCOLATE SWISS ROLL «

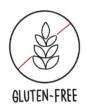

GLUTEN-FREE

serves 10

DOUGH

3/4 cup almond flour

3/4 cup oat flour

10 Medjool dates, pitted

1/4 cup cacao powder

1/2 tsp ground vanilla bean

2-3 Tbsp water

COCO WHIP

1 can full fat coconut cream (the solid part)

1 Tbsp maple syrup

1/2 tsp vanilla extract

COATING

300gr dark vegan chocolate, melted

desiccated coconut

With a crunchy chocolate shell on the outside, a soft chocolate dough beneath and a creamy coconut filling, this chocolate swiss roll makes the perfect combination for a heavenly treat!

1. For the dough, simply place all the ingredients in a high-speed blender and mix until smooth. Line a square baking tin (8" x 8") with parchment paper.
2. Spread the dough evenly in the tin, pressing down with your fingers. Place in your freezer for 10 minutes.
3. Prepare the coconut whip by scooping out only the firm part of cream from the can and placing it in a chilled bowl. Add the remaining ingredients and use a mixer to whip it up.
4. Take out the dough from the freezer, take it out of the tin with the parchment paper and evenly spread the coconut whip on top.
5. Slowly start rolling up the dough from one side until you have a firm roll. Place the roll back into the freezer and melt your chocolate.
6. Pour the chocolate over the roll, add toppings and let it dry. Let sit at room temperature for 5 minutes before eating!

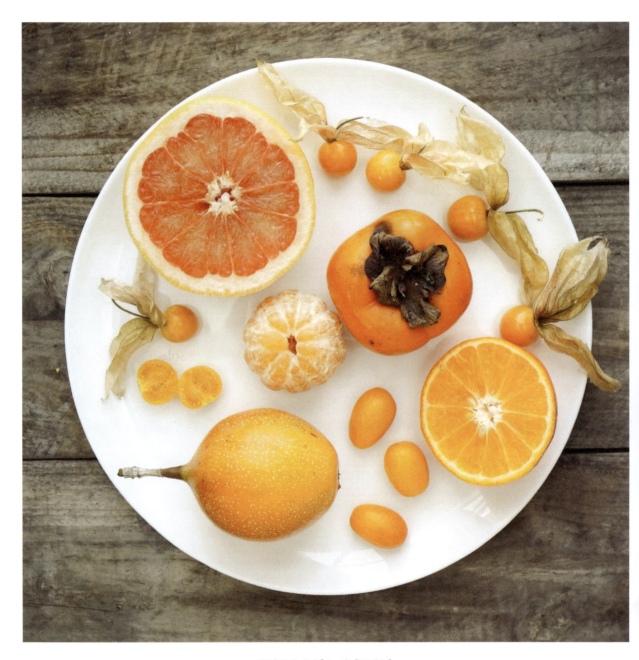

THANK YOU!

•••

Thank you so much for supporting me!
Thanks to your contribution I can continue creating both delicious AND healthy recipes for you on 'The Tasty K', as well as publish new cook books that will hopefully inspire you on your journey to a healthy lifestyle!

ACKNOWLEDGEMENTS

Disclaimers

The use of the website www.thetastyk.com and this publication is at the sole risk of the reader. The book is designed to give information and inspiration to our readers and not intended to replace medical advice. No warranties or guarantees are expressed or implied in the content of the information provided.

The author expressly disclaims responsability for any adverese effects arising from following advice given in this book without appropriate medical supervision. You accept all risks and responsability for losses, damages, costs and other consequences resulting directly or indirectly from using this site and any information or material available from it.

The recipes in this book have been created for the ingredients and techniques indicated. Any modifications to suit your dietary requirements may result in change of taste or texture.

Attributions

Photography: Kirsten Kaminski & Ana-Christina Fluieras
Design and production: Kirsten Kaminski & Daniel Rechter
Sources and information: www.nutritionfacts.org

Printed in Poland
by Amazon Fulfillment
Poland Sp. z o.o., Wrocław

36307468R00049